Prioritizing Health and Well-Being

Prioritizing Health and Well-Being

Self-Care as a Leadership Strategy for School Leaders

Brian K. Creasman

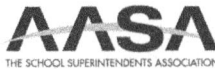

AASA
THE SCHOOL SUPERINTENDENTS ASSOCIATION

ROWMAN & LITTLEFIELD
Lanham • Boulder • New York • London

AASA
THE SCHOOL SUPERINTENDENTS ASSOCIATION

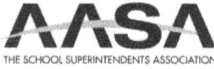

Published in conjunction with AASA

Published by Rowman & Littlefield
An imprint of The Rowman & Littlefield Publishing Group, Inc.
4501 Forbes Boulevard, Suite 200, Lanham, Maryland 20706
www.rowman.com

86-90 Paul Street, London EC2A 4NE

British Library Cataloguing in Publication Information Available

Library of Congress Cataloging-in-Publication Data

Names: Creasman, Brian, author.
Title: Prioritizing health and well-being : self-care as a leadership strategy for school
    leaders / Brian K. Creasman.
Description: Lanham : Rowman & Littlefield, [2022] | Includes bibliographical
    references. | Summary: "The superintendency requires an elevated level of stamina
    due to the complexities superintendents face each day. Through both personal and
    professional perspectives, Prioritizing Health and Well-Being places emphasis on the
    career of superintendents in terms of prioritizing health and well-being to remain
    effective in their leadership journey"— Provided by publisher.
Identifiers: LCCN 2022023241 (print) | LCCN 2022023242 (ebook) | ISBN
    9781475867367 (cloth) | 9781475867374 (paper) | ISBN 9781475867381 (ebook)
Subjects: LCSH: School superintendents—Job stress. | School superintendents—
    Mental health. | School management and organization—Psychological aspects. |
    Educational leadership.
Classification: LCC LB2831.73 .C74 2022 (print) | LCC LB2831.73 (ebook) |
    DDC 371.2/011—dc23/eng/20220706
LC record available at https://lccn.loc.gov/2022023241
LC ebook record available at https://lccn.loc.gov/2022023242

To Valerie and Georgia,
Thank you both for your love and support and for
helping me find a healthier work-life balance.
I love you both!

Contents

Foreword

The position of superintendent has gotten more complex over the decades. This has been recognized both anecdotally as well as through research (Brunner, Grogan, & Bjork, 2002; Carter & Cunningham, 1997; Kowalski, 2005). The No Child Left Behind Act of 2001 added new pressures associated with the accountability movement. While high-stakes testing and accountability are still a constant presence within a school district, additional pressures also grew with funding shortages, school choice and vouchers, and the rise of social media, to name a few.

All of these competing responsibilities and the nonstop nature of the position are often mentioned when determining the amount of stress a superintendent is experiencing in the position. The School Superintendents Association (AASA) has conducted decade studies allowing for a longitudinal look at the position. One area—the level of stress—has continued to grow over time.

In 1980, 43.6 percent of superintendents reported being highly stressed. This percentage increased to 51.5 percent in 2000 (Glass & Franceschini, 2007). This percentage increased again to 61 percent in the latest 2020 decennial survey (Tienken, 2021). While this inquiry is just one question of a much larger survey, it is worth noting that there is not a lot of research on the topic of superintendent stress. Most often, the topic is addressed through dissertations (Kane, 2017; Peterson, 2017; Targgart, 2017).

In 2015, Charol Shakeshaft and I decided to conduct a national study looking more closely at superintendent stress and health. The resulting article, "Superintendent Stress and Superintendent Health: A National Study," found that while superintendents did experience stress, it often wasn't as severe as previously reported. What was more alarming was the finding that there was a meaningful relationship between day-to-day stress and the number of health conditions developed while serving as a superintendent (Robinson & Shakeshaft, 2016).

While there were findings highlighting the issues with stress and its effect on a superintendent's health, this wasn't the entire story. One benefit of the open-ended component of the survey allowed for participants to provide more insight into their experiences. While a number of respondents shared about their medical issues, others highlighted taking care of themselves as a priority, and the impact it had on their overall health. It was stories like these, focusing on well-being and flourishing, that we were excited to explore next in a qualitative follow-up study.

And then 2020 happened. As if the superintendency wasn't challenging enough, the past two years have brought a whole new level of trials and issues that require immediate and ongoing focus. The COVID-19 pandemic, issues of systemic racism, virtual and hybrid learning, vaccine requirements, critical race theory, mask debates, and book banning all were thrust onto center stage in very public ways.

Social media amplified these topics, often highlighting the extremes, all of which superintendents needed to navigate, and often operating in a no-win situation. Additionally, public protests and unruly behavior at school board meetings became regular occurrences in districts across the country. The anger and vitriol were often directed right at the superintendents. Instead of the public recognizing the ongoing planning focused on care and support that was being offered during this tumultuous time filled with multiple pivots, most narratives focused on the negatives. Was this already complex position just becoming too cumbersome? Would there be a mass exodus with leaders abandoning the superintendency?

While some superintendents have found this to be an ideal time to leave the position, thankfully, most are committed to remain and continue the important work they do for their districts each day. Additionally, others continue to aspire to the superintendency, not letting the current landscape deter them from pursuing this vital position. One thing that helps both sitting and aspiring superintendents is identifying avenues of support. This may come from mentors, formal and informal networks, professional learning opportunities, as well as resources targeted specifically for the superintendency.

This is where Brian's book comes into play. *Prioritizing Health and Well-Being* provides insights from a sitting superintendent about the importance of filling up your own cup before sharing with others. The field of education is one of service, and for most in the superintendency, it often equates to many years of putting others first. This book gives you permission to pause and focus on yourself by listening to what your body is trying to tell you.

Prioritizing Health and Well-Being provides fantastic insights to help keep you grounded as you work with the complexities of the job. The advice is practical and achievable with wonderful strategies provided throughout, as well as embedded "Voices from the Field" within each chapter that share the experiences of superintendents. While the book can be read sequentially from front to back, I also love that each chapter provides a particular focus that can be read in isolation.

For example, after a particularly challenging day, superintendents may choose to turn to the chapter "Never Lose Hope or Abandon Your Dreams" to help them remember their why. The book concludes with an appendix containing fifteen strategies to help prioritize health and well-being as a perfect means to jumpstart the practice of focusing on yourself first. While the idea of "putting the oxygen mask on yourself first" may not be something a superintendent is used to doing, it is vital for both short-term and long-term health and well-being and for the ability to remain committed to the students, families, and communities you serve.

Kerry Robinson, PhD
University of North Carolina Wilmington

Preface

"The journey of a thousand miles begins with one step."

—Lao Tzu

Almost every book that I have coauthored begins with an introduction where the coauthors and I state that we try to stay away from educational jargon that plagues most books about education, no matter whether it was a focus on teacher leadership, leadership networks, school transformation, or communication. This book is no different. Although I author it alone, I want to stay away from educational jargon or well-being jargon. This is a book about a personal topic through a leadership perspective, specifically the superintendency.

I have been so fortunate in my career to learn, collaborate, and work with so many phenomenal students, teachers, staff, and school administrators in Georgia, North Carolina, and now Kentucky. I work for a phenomenal Board of Education and live in a student-first community. Furthermore, through my network of colleagues that stretches throughout the nation and globe, I have also learned what to do, but more importantly what not to do. One former North Carolina superintendent who is not a national consultant, said, "Brian, you can get another superintendency, but you can't ever get a new body. If you fail to focus on your well-being, your superintendency will never be what it could be." How correct he was.

If I could turn back time, like Cher, and do things differently as an assistant principal, principal, assistant superintendent, I would have made well-being a priority. Though my journey of discovering the importance of well-being has taken fifteen years, at least I have come to realize the importance. As you read this book, think about how many superintendents are behind desks who have no clue that the clock is ticking on their well-being and, therefore, their superintendency. Though no one is promised tomorrow, we can improve our chances by finding a healthy work-life balance.

For full transparency, in life and at work, I have missed so many opportunities. Though I would like to think I have changed the lives of so many, I always think about those that I couldn't help or accidentally missed or overlooked. What if I had made their well-being a priority instead of something else, like curriculum, test scores, after-school faculty/staff meetings, that education says are the most important things? What if I saw them as authentically human?

Education is a profession focused on people, yet in too many cases we fail people all the time. We have made "well-doing" a priority over "well-being" for far too long. We care more about end-of-year high-stakes testing, instead of student disengagement and teacher burnout. We have met the enemy and it is us, educators and educational leaders, who see test data but overlook the person. Leadership is more about the little things and less about the big things. Few people will remember leaders for what they accomplish, but instead, how they treat people.

Prioritizing Health and Well-Being is personal to me, and I try to offer relevant strategies on how to make health and well-being part of the superintendency. As I wrote each day for almost two years, I had to stop so many times because of things that would make me think. With each word, I offer a reflection of something that I discovered was missing in my life—well-being. *Prioritizing Health and Well-Being* is inherently a human story about a superintendent who has the best job in Kentucky, a great family, who struggles each day finding a balance between work and life. I have failed so many times, but through each failure, I discover new paths, and I hope they help you.

Purpose

> "Wellbeing is about the combination of our love for what we do each day, the quality of our relationships, the security of our finances, the vibrancy of our physical health, and the pride we take in what we love contributed to our communities. Most importantly, it's about how these five elements interact." –Tim Rath

The purpose of *Prioritizing Health and Well-Being* is to shed light on the importance of self-care for superintendents. The importance of self-care has received a lot of focus over the past several years, especially among students and educators. Though educators' self-care is important and widely discussed, often the health and well-being of superintendents is overlooked and has not been fully discussed or documented. *Prioritizing Health and Well-Being* walks current superintendents, assistant superintendents/directors, as well as aspiring superintendents through key strategies to bring self-care to the forefront in their important leadership position.

Self-care should not be seen as a standalone strategy but something embedded into daily practice. In fact, to make health and well-being a priority, both self-care and the superintendency must be interwoven together in such a way that superintendents develop a high level of awareness of their own well-being and see it as critical to their overall effectiveness as a leader.

Too often, superintendents focus so much time on many traditional components of the job, such as teaching and learning, the budget, day-to-day operations, accountability, community involvement and partnerships, and the well-being of others. In doing so, they push their own well-being to the backburner. Since the early spring of 2020, the pressures of the superintendents have increased exponentially because of the global health pandemic (COVID-19), social justice movements, cultural wars, and political differences. Therefore, well-being must be made a priority and practiced daily to counteract these new demands, pressures, and stressors.

Superintendents have become more tense and stressed over the past couple of years, which is why superintendents are retiring or leaving the profession in search of new jobs and professions at alarming rates. Education remains the most important job in the world, as educators teach tomorrow's educators, leaders, attorneys, physicians, and superintendents. Yet, right now, the job of the superintendency has lost some of the attraction, because of how easily it can consume the life of the person.

There must be a major shift not just in education but also in the superintendency. The rate of turnover and retirement of superintendents is not sustainable at its current level. As superintendents leave the position, a vacuum forms by pulling directors and principals to fill superintendent vacancies, which in turn creates additional vacancies, adding to the national shortage of principals and teachers. It is mission-critical to transform the superintendency by prioritizing the leader's health. No leader can be effective, at least not for long, with poor health or well-being.

The goal of *Prioritizing Health and Well-Being* is to bring awareness to the importance of health and well-being with the hope of spreading across the school district, positively impacting teachers, staff, and, yes, students. Superintendents must model the way with well-being, just like with everything they else are responsible for. In education, self-care is often discussed in terms of students, teachers, and staff, but it is just as important for leadership positions.

At this point, education requires a transformative moment where well-being becomes the priority. Gone are the days of the mindset of well-being being optional. Without a priority on health and well-being, all the priorities at the end seem futile because the overall effectiveness or success of each one requires long-term leadership capacity, which requires a healthy work-life balance by superintendents.

In more concise terms, *Prioritizing Health and Well-Being* is a call to action for superintendents to take back their health so that they can lead their school districts more effectively and for the long term. School districts, students, teachers, boards of education, and communities need leaders who are committed for the long term. The rising turnover rate of superintendents is alarming and not sustainable. The turnover rate, because of increasing burnout, is impacting the effectiveness of school districts for the short and long terms. Right now, school districts need stability at the top, and superintendents finding the appropriate and effective work-life balance would be a great first step.

Students, teachers, parents, and the community need a superintendent's leadership right now during this critical educational moment. With so much unrest and uncertainty, school districts and communities need the chief educational officer to lead. Though health and well-being are inherently personal, superintendents making their health and well-being a priority in their lives and work each day will change the lives of hundreds, if not thousands. Superintendents must prioritize their health and well-being if they expect to be effective leaders for the long haul and have quality of life during retirement.

How Did Superintendents Overlook the Importance of their Well-Being?

"There are times when it will go so wrong that you will be barely alive, and times when you realize that being barely alive, on your own terms, is better than living a bloated half-life on someone else's terms."
—Jeanette Winterson

The many demands of the superintendency are nothing to take lightly. Until you have sat in the superintendent's chair, you can't begin to fathom the job or . . . the calling. From the time superintendents enter their graduate program, seldom is health and well-being ever mentioned. Superintendents are trained to keep going no matter the circumstance. In simple terms, superintendents are trained and, in some cases, encouraged to go to the point of physical breakdown and mental exhaustion.

Early mornings, late evenings, weekend office hours, short vacations, and no time for themselves over the past half-century, have resulted in epidemic burnout of superintendents today. As leaders, superintendents are trained to focus on themselves last, compromising their own health for the sake of others. The logic behind the notion that leaders must eat last overlooks the importance of health and well-being. If superintendents expect to be effective professionally, their health must be a priority.

Over the past half-century, society has created a system in education in which those who work eighty hours a week end up with short tenures as superintendents, are somewhat celebrated for sacrificing their body, mind, and spirit, while penalizing those superintendents who work fewer hours, focus on their health, and have longer tenures. The "system" rewards superintendents who never take vacations or spend time with family but eventually burn out, while penalizing the superintendents who have created a healthy work-life balance. In other words, superintendents have become a victim of an outdated system that they created!

The system created is not forgiving and is still primarily designed for the following demographic: old, Caucasian, and male. Though over the past five years the superintendency has increased in diversity, bringing in more superintendents of color, younger superintendents, and female superintendents, the system is still shackled to yesterday, not tomorrow. That system, the superintendency, still expects superintendents to give everything, even if it includes sacrificing their own health and well-being. As a result, superintendents are leaving the profession because of burnout or retirement at an alarming rate that quite simply is not sustainable for the long term.

Though the turnover rate of superintendents is high, and the average tenure is only three to five years, there is no indication that change is happening, leading to even more burnout of superintendents. Right now, the superintendency is designed to work men and women to the point of burnout and, unfortunately, to death in many circumstances. Speak to a superintendent today and more than likely they know someone, a colleague, who passed away while a superintendent. This is heartbreaking and jarring. The job expects the superintendent to give everything, sacrificing their health and family. But it doesn't have to be this way. To be clear, the superintendency hasn't been healthy for anyone over the past fifty years, no matter what people may think.

Yes, fifty years ago, superintendents may have stayed on the job longer, but that doesn't mean they had a better or healthier work-life balance. The superintendency from yesteryear was starkly different from what superintendents face today. Fifty years ago, people didn't recognize the importance of health and well-being in their relationship to their job. If they did recognize it, they knew not to speak about it. Today is different. The superintendency is hemorrhaging men and women each day. All the while, few of quality are standing in line to step into these vacancies.

There is an urgent need to figure out what is happening in the superintendency today. Boards of education have dramatically changed over the past fifty years. Most boards of education expect superintendents to take care of their health, even though superintendents remain fixated on working long hours, taking no time off, spending less time with family, and spending little time on their own health and well-being. There is no benefit to boards of education with a constant carousel of superintendents.

Though the superintendency is demanding, it is also rewarding. Superintendents have an excellent opportunity to change the trajectory of the profession going forward. There must be a clear understanding that to be an effective leader, the leader's well-being must be the priority. No leader can lead effectively if their health and well-being are compromised. If they can, by luck, they don't lead for too long. When there is a misalignment between the job and well-being, the leader's health and well-being impairment unfortunately eventually costs the leader too much of everything.

Superintendents don't have to continue to cling to an outdated model that is only exacerbating the number of superintendents who are exhausted and leaving the profession for health reasons. The job will still be demanding, but superintendents must equip themselves with the understanding that their health and well-being are the priority and strategy to effectiveness and longevity.

It doesn't matter how many preparation programs superintendents have successfully completed or the number of degrees they have earned; if health and well-being aren't made a priority, their tenure will be short. The future of the superintendency doesn't look too promising, but that can change. The job doesn't have to continue to be shackled to the requirements of half a century ago. Superintendents must begin to communicate the importance of their own health and well-being regarding the success of the district and the health and well-being of students, teachers, bus drivers, and other staff members.

If the superintendent is not healthy, then the district's culture cannot be healthy. Superintendents must model the way, and that starts with their own health and well-being, leading others and making them understand the importance of their health and well-being. No one can ever go wrong with prioritizing their health and well-being; however, they can go very wrong if they fail to do so.

At the end of the day, that is what superintendents face today. For far too long, superintendents have failed to make their own health and well-being a focus or priority. Those superintendents suffered, compromising their own health, and in some cases losing everything their health, families, and friends. Just because the history of the superintendency may appear grim with respect to a leader's health, it doesn't mean the future can't look different. The only requirement is that superintendents today make a course correction, communicate, and model the importance of health and well-being.

The Why Behind Self-Care

"Self-care is not self-indulgence, it is self-preservation."

—Audre Lorde

It may be hard to believe, but sometimes the why behind something must be spelled out clearly, in relevant terms, so that the reader may fully understand the importance. A superintendent's health and well-being are two terms that must be spelled out clearly. Though superintendents may understand what the words mean, most struggle with prioritizing both. Each day, as the superintendency becomes more difficult and overwhelming, the level of stress is certain to increase as well.

Since the start of the global pandemic caused by COVID-19 in the early spring of 2020, health and well-being have become a buzzword throughout education. Though everyone is talking and writing about health and well-being, this focus has not translated into system-wide practice among educators, including superintendents. Superintendents recognize the need to prioritize their health and well-being, but most continue to struggle to balance that with the requirements of the job.

If one performs a search on the Internet with any of these words or phrases—"superintendent well-being," "superintendent health", or "superintendent self-care strategies"—or any phrase relating to the superintendency, health, self-care, and well-being, they may be shocked to learn that few resources are available that directly focus on superintendent health and well-being.

Superintendents, like everyone, need not only to be encouraged to make health and well-being a priority but also to evaluate how it looks in their day-to-day personal and professional lives. Most people can't imagine not working nonstop, taking breaks to meditate, eating healthy, or exercising

xx   ∼   Preface

daily. They believe that they are "too far gone" to make course corrections, but that is not correct.

It is never too late for superintendents to make their own health and well-being a priority. Though a superintendent may be late into their career, on the downhill, close to retirement, they still can make changes in their life that will add years and improve their quality of life, while in the office and post-superintendency. The goal is for superintendents to realize this early in their careers so that they have time to make necessary course corrections. Change is not easy but can be done.

Throughout this book, key topics are presented with practical strategies. They can be used by the novice or veteran superintendent, who may also be new to prioritizing their health and well-being. No matter where the superintendent may be in their career, the strategies presented offer practical options for everyone. The strategies offered are not rocket science, but practical and meaningful strategies and suggestions that can be easily adopted—whether individually or collectively.

Ultimately, like with most things, superintendents are responsible for their own health and well-being. Superintendents, in their positions, have control over so much. Though no matter how much superintendents try to control, most practice little control in prioritizing their own health. When asked, superintendents will have a variety of excuses as to why they can't seem to focus on their health, ranging from schedule conflicts to a lack of expertise. Few, if any, superintendents will say they don't see the importance of their health or well-being.

With superintendents and their health and well-being, both must be tangible, flexible, and relevant to their lives and jobs. This book is important, as all the strategies given can be adapted to each superintendent's situation, schedule, and goals. Though time is a valuable commodity with superintendents, every superintendent must be available for their own health and well-being.

The well-being of students, teachers, and the staff depends on how effective a leader is at prioritizing their own well-being. Like with most everything else, scheduling and time-management resides with the superintendent. He or she must choose whether to make time for their health and well-being or not. No one else can do that for them. If the superintendent struggles with their health and well-being, others do as well. At the end of the day, self-care is intimately personal, but as a superintendent, your own self-care prioritize has huge positive implications for others. Superintendents lead and model the way for others along the self-care journey.

Acknowledgments

The job of superintendents grows more difficult with each passing day. Though the job isn't for the faint of heart, it is one of the most rewarding jobs in the nation. Superintendents across the nation have a direct or indirect impact on student outcomes, staff success, and community support in one form or another. Superintendents are critical to the overall success of public education, the economy, and the nation's prosperity. However, many overlook the importance of superintendents.

In the pages of *Prioritizing Health and Well-Being*, I have learned so much about superintendency, not about the normal areas of focus but on the personal side of the superintendency. Each superintendency, no matter the size of the school district, involves a human being who gives everything that they have, including their health and well-being, to a very demanding job.

To be effective, superintendents must be committed to, not just involved in, leadership. As I wrote *Prioritizing Health and Well-Being*, I had the opportunity to speak with hundreds of superintendents across the nation—from Maine to Hawaii, Alaska to Florida, and every state in between. It has been a journey of two years to make sure to identify the most practical, right, and aligned information for superintendents pertaining to health and well-being.

Health and well-being aren't something that a superintendent achieves; it is not a destination but instead a journey and ongoing continuous improvement process. Health and well-being require an ongoing day-to-day focus and long-term commitment from each individual. Though both are not achieved overnight, the process is not as complicated as many believe. At the end of the day, neither take fancy programs, extreme amounts of time, or expensive equipment.

As I will mention in chapter 1, the three most transformative things a person can do for their health and well-being are to drink water, get a good night's sleep, and exercise at least three to four times each week (especially by walking). All three are free but elusive to so many, including superintendents. As I learned through interviewing, researching, and writing, at the end of the day, time was the common theme that continued to be the obstacle superintendents struggled to get around. Repeatedly, I heard from current and former superintendents, in one form or another, "I don't have time . . . to drink water, sleep, or exercise."

Throughout *Prioritizing Health and Well-Being*, examples (Practical Strategies) and stories (Voices from the Field) are provided to offer the reader real experiences from current and former superintendents in an effort to show that creating a healthy work-life balance is possible. I would be remiss if I failed to thank the hundreds of superintendents, physicians, nutritionists, fitness trainers, and other health experts who spoke to me as I was doing background research for the book. There are too many to mention, and I would undoubtedly forget someone. The superintendents, physicians, nutritionists, fitness trainers, and other health experts know who they are, and I hope I was able to bring their contributions to life in the pages that follow.

The recommendations on the back cover are from some of the most recognizable leaders in the nation today. They are leaders, writers, mentors, practitioners, and, more importantly, friends, to whom I am indebted for their help. I want to thank Wayne Lewis, Jack Hoke, Mike Lubelfeld, Nick Polyak, and Rob Jackson for their early review of the book and their kind and powerful words that help to stress just how important self-care is to superintendents and leaders in today's schools.

This book is the culmination of a two-year process that at times I did not think I could finish. Just as many superintendents feel focusing on their health and well-being is difficult, trying to find the right information to share proved to be equally difficult. But I want to thank Phil Eason, a leadership consultant and former superintendent, who constantly reminded me just how important health and well-being are to leaders. He provided valuable feedback on chapters. Phil is an excellent leader who helps other leaders focus on what matters the most. One of my favorite quotes that Phil uses regularly is, "We (education) have been focused too long on the well-doing and not enough on the well-being." Not only is Phil a leadership consultant, he has been an excellent mentor and friend since 2019. Each week our virtual conversations, emails, and texts are invaluable to me personally and professionally.

To make this book meaningful for superintendents (aspiring, novice, or veteran) I needed to find two leaders and practitioners who could bring health and well-being into focus. When I sought individuals to write the foreword and afterword, I tried to identify practitioners in the field, innovative leaders, or recognizable names in the field of education. Luckily, two of the most recognizable innovative leaders and practitioners agreed to help without question.

Dr. Kerry Robinson, assistant professor and MSA program coordinator in the Department of Education Leadership at UNC Wilmington, started the book in the foreword with the level of urgency self-care demands. Her work and advocacy around superintendent self-care are recognized across the nation. Few research studies have been conducted about superintendent self-care, but Kerry is one of the researchers who conducted a nationwide study that still is widely used by superintendent preparation programs and superintendent trainings. Kerry, your foreword is everything I hoped it would be and much more.

The afterword was written by Dr. Susan Enfield, superintendent of Highline Public Schools in Washington. Susan is a nationwide leader who other superintendents follow. Her reputation as an advocate for students is the gold standard for superintendents across the nation. Her vast experience in public education is simply unparalleled in the circle of district leadership today. When she speaks, other leaders listen, which is why she is often found facilitating and leading nationwide discussions in public education today. Her advocacy is the beacon for others to follow. Susan, your leadership and advocacy shined through once again and provided the path forward for the superintendency.

One of the most important sections of the book is the "Call to Action" written by Dan Domenech, executive director of AASA. Dan, through his career, has worked with thousands of superintendents nationwide and internationally. His advocacy for public education will never be matched again in our lifetimes. When presidents or secretaries of education need advice about public education they call Dan, which speaks to his extensive career, exceptional advocacy, and leadership.

In the "Call to Action," Dan encourages every superintendent to take notice of just how important their health and well-being are to their success as a school leader. Equally as important, Dan stresses that a superintendent's health has a direct impact on the health of the school district. In other words, a culture of health and well-being starts at the top. Dan, thank you for once again helping to frame just how important the superintendency is today.

I also want to acknowledge two individuals who are important partners behind the scenes, Tom Koerner, vice president and senior executive editor of the Education Divison at Rowman & Littlefield Publishers, and James "Jimmy" Minichello, director of communications and public relations at AASA. Thank you for responding to my many emails and text messages. Also, thank you both for supporting my ideas and helping me bring each book to fruition. Neither gets recognized enough, but they are cheerleaders in the background, encouraging authors, and are equally excited with each book published. Thank you.

Like superintendents, boards of education, since March 2020, have endured an unimaginable onslaught of complaints and criticisms. I am so grateful to the Fleming County Board of Education for giving me the opportunity of a lifetime to work in Fleming County Schools. Thank you for your continued support and for your work to ensure every student has an opportunity to succeed. I do have the best job in Kentucky!

Lastly, but certainly not least, I want to acknowledge my wife, Valerie, and my daughter, Georgia. Both are so important to me, though they, like many superintendents' families, often take a backseat to the demands of the job. Over the past two years as I wrote this book, I tried to practice what I wrote and have spent more time with them—that I will always treasure. I am blessed to have both in my life. I am also so proud of each one of them for their achievements, Valerie for being an awesome school counselor and Georgia for being an eight-year-old gymnast and full-of-life artist. Thank you both for everything that you both do and for allowing me to do what I love doing.

Writer Acknowledgment

A Call to Action by
Daniel A. Domenech
Executive Director
AASA, The School Superintendents Association

Afterword by
Dr. Susan Enfield
Superintendent
Highline Public Schools, Washington

A Call to Action

Hardly a day goes by when I don't receive a call from a reporter asking me to share my thoughts about the unprecedented number of superintendents who have chosen to retire from their positions. I've been in this business for more than half a century, and I have never seen anything like it. To compound the problem, as top-notch educators are stepping down from the profession, individuals lacking the essential experience are moving into leadership positions.

As I noted in my column in the September 2021 issue of *School Administrator* magazine, we're hearing from scores of superintendents who are leaving their posts, not because of retirement or relocation to other districts, but because of the stress created by the pandemic and related factors. To make matters worse, superintendents and their families are being physically threatened. We are trying to navigate through what is now the third academic year of the COVID-19 pandemic.

The current environment has impacted all aspects of how we educate our children, from attendance to instruction to transportation to mask mandates to the homework gap to staffing to resource inequities and much more. When I'm not Zooming, I'm on the phone with superintendents on a continuing basis about these sensitive topics. Grinding through an avalanche of crises requires unparalleled leadership, which is why I could not be more proud of these "Champions for Children," as I call them, who are working diligently every single day to fight for equity and the safety and welfare of the children in their respective school communities.

If there is one thing that is certain in a world full of unpleasantries and uncertainties like we find ourselves in today, it's this: every school-system leader, administrator, building leader, lead teacher, or anyone associated with educating our children needs to raise the bar when it comes to self-care. My friend Brian Creasman, the 2020 Kentucky Superintendent of the Year, is spot on by urging superintendents, through the pages of this book, to make self-health and self-care a huge priority. I was a superintendent for nearly thirty years, and I can tell you the job is tough enough. If we don't take care of ourselves, how can we expect to do the job effectively?

AASA is doing its part. At a time when school system leaders need our support more than ever, we recently launched "Live Well. Lead Well."—a campaign focused on supporting the health and well-being of our school leaders.

Paul Imhoff, superintendent of Ohio's Upper Arlington Schools and the 2021–2022 president, initiated the campaign. He once said, "Students who aren't well, can't learn. Teachers who aren't well, can't teach. Leaders who aren't well, can't lead. We need to take care of ourselves so that we can serve those in our care. We can't lead if we aren't well." Can anyone dispute any of these statements?

As part of the campaign, we are featuring monthly webinars that focus on self-care, student-care, and staff-care, as well as leadership changes and bringing communities back together. Our campaign is about providing superintendents and their staffs with the tools and resources they need to help ease stressors of the job, support their important work, show appreciation for their leadership, and fuel their spirit to keep them moving forward.

Brian points out that if a superintendent does not become a model for self-care, how can we expect staff, faculty, families, and students to do so? As we move forward, we're getting closer and closer to what will eventually become the other side of the pandemic. Whether you're an educator or not, please heed the words you read in *Prioritizing Health and Well-Being*. Do it for yourself and for all of those around you. Set the example, and become the model.

Our schools and communities depend on it. The future of our children is at stake.

Daniel A. Domenech
Executive Director
AASA, The School Superintendents Association

Introduction

"I think a hero is an ordinary individual who finds the strength to persevere and endure despite overwhelming obstacles."
—Christopher Reeve

Prioritizing Health and Well-Being provides superintendents with practical well-being strategies. Well-being over the past several years has gained attention. Increasing advertisements, commercials, research, textbooks, webinars, conferences, self-help books, and many other informational pieces and events have brought well-being into a daily topic in education. With the onset of COVID-19 back in the early spring of 2020, well-being became a more heavily discussed topic as the terms "underlying health condition" were mentioned daily in the news.

Even in 2022, few school leaders have come to realize the importance of well-being. There is nothing easy about maintaining a healthy well-being. It takes work and patience, and never consists of overnight successes. Well-being is a marathon that requires stamina and a destination. *Prioritizing Health and Well-Being* introduces school superintendents to the importance of their health and its impact on their leadership.

Leaders must establish a pace that they can maintain over the long term. There will be roadblocks, obstacles, and failures throughout the marathon. They must push through, go around, pick themselves up, and keep moving forward. Their families, students, staff, and communities need their health and well-being to be good. Health and well-being are not things to overlook, especially for superintendents who face increasing stress.

Prioritizing Health and Well-Being is about helping superintendents recognize the importance of well-being in terms of increasing their longevity as a superintendent. Though written through the lens of a superintendent, this book provides practical strategies for all educational leaders and even those leaders who may lead large and dynamic organizations, such as a school or school district. *Prioritizing Health and Well-Being* offers practical strategies for the aspiring, novice, or most veteran superintendent.

What is conveyed throughout *Prioritizing Health and Well-Being* is that it is never too late to focus on well-being. With the complexities superintendents face today and will continue to face going forward, all superintendents are encouraged to begin now. If they decide to start tomorrow that is fine, the key is to take the first step to become a better leader. In other words, health and well-being require action at some point. No matter if the superintendent is out of shape or the fittest leader, they must take the first step in the growth process.

Superintendents model the way for others in so many ways. Superintendents are instructional leaders, athletic leaders, business leaders, public relations leaders, and community leaders. In recent years, many superintendents have taken on the title of chief learner—meaning they model the way to embrace each day as a learning opportunity. In many respects, superintendents are students themselves on multiple levels—learning something new each day.

But what if superintendents became chief well-being officers, CWOs, modeling the way for everyone in the district to start the journey to a healthier well-being. The thing about a chief well-being officer is that by focusing on well-being, they touch so many other facets found within the district, including learning, performance, and community outreach. Who better to be the well-being leader for the community since stakeholders look to the superintendent for so many other things?

It is not hard to believe that students, teachers, staff, boards of education, and the community need and want a superintendent who is healthy. It does no district any good when the superintendent changes year to year or every three to five years. All school districts need superintendents who are there for the long term. More importantly, students, the primary focus of education, need a district leader who models the way and cares about their well-being, not just their test scores.

Look at the districts that have been fortunate to have superintendents who have long tenures in the district, and chances are you will find stability, high student performance, increased parent and community engagement, and a healthy leader. A veteran superintendent, with longevity in the same office, is most likely healthy. Well-being requires a strategy, not a coincidence. Unfortunately, no one happens to wish their way to fitness, health, or well-being.

Prioritizing Health and Well-Being tries to correct the wrong of many decades in education through the superintendency. There are no groundbreaking ideas, solutions to high-stakes testing, or closing the achievement gap offered within these pages. No, the goal is to start a conversation about the health gap that is not only crippling education but the nation's economic, military, and academic strength each day. This growing health and well-being gap must become a national security focus, not solely a topic mentioned in schools and school districts. A tsunami of catastrophic proportions is forming on the horizon. Superintendents must stop just for a few minutes to think about their quality of health, as well as the well-being of students, teachers, and staff.

If superintendents are not focused on well-being, who else in the school district will make well-being a priority. Newsflash, the superintendent is the gatekeeper to well-being. If the superintendent fails to find value in well-being, then the health of the organization will never be healthy. Likewise, the well-being of students, teachers, and staff will never be made a priority. In today's society of rapidly increasing sedentary students, obese students and staff, and increasing premature deaths, public education must take the lead before it's too late.

Superintendents do so many wonderful things each day, except taking care of their well-being. If teachers need textbooks, superintendents are there calling to find the textbook and appropriating the funds to purchase the textbooks. But on the other side, if the superintendent is struggling with sleeping at night due to stress, we simply brush it aside and chalk it up to the pressures of the job. It doesn't have to be this way.

Though we tell ourselves we are working hard, speeding to the edges of death, for students, we are not helping them like we think we are. As mentioned earlier, what students need the most is a superintendent who will be there for them, value them, and care about their well-being. In truly clear terms, no superintendent can help someone else if they are not taking care of themselves first.

Superintendents, assistant superintendents, aspiring superintendents, directors, and principals are in a race against time. Now is the time for superintendents to take the lead, gain an understanding of the importance of health and well-being, and change the culture going forward. Together superintendents can transform education by focusing on the health of the organization through their own well-being and the well-being of their students, teachers, and staff. For far too long, educators, principals, and superintendents have been focused on "well-doing" and not on "well-being."

How *Prioritizing Health and Well-Being* Is Organized

Prioritizing Health and Well-Being places an emphasis on the career of superintendents in terms of prioritizing their health and well-being to remain effective in their leadership journey. The superintendency today requires an elevated level of stamina due to the complexities superintendents face each day. The book addresses the critical importance of health and well-being, while also improving their overall effectiveness as a leader as a way to navigate the job of being the chief executive of the district.

Structure
Prioritizing Health and Well-Being is divided up into twenty-two chapters. The reader will be able to use each chapter individually or all together, based on where they may be in their leadership journey. At the beginning of each chapter, the reader is provided an opening quote, followed by an introduction. Each chapter contains a section dedicated to Practical Strategies. The Voices from the Field capture real stories about self-care from current or former superintendents. At the end of each chapter, the reader is invited to review a critical Takeaway for each chapter before moving to the next chapter.

Finding a healthy work-life balance is critical for superintendents' longevity. Too many superintendents are retiring or leaving the profession at an alarming rate due to exhaustion, burnout, or diminished health. In other words, the pressure of the job has become too great, and few have strategies to counteract this daunting and, in some cases, debilitating job. Likewise, too many superintendents who are fortunate to retire live a confining life due to overall poor health.

Based on research, no book has specifically focused solely on superintendents' health and well-being. Most books have only, at most, designated a chapter about the self-care of superintendents. *Prioritizing Health and Well-Being* seeks to fill the void in research and practical tools for superintendents. Endurance is based on my years of experience. This book provides real strategies, based on experiences, to validate the importance of self-care as mission-critical to superintendents' effectiveness and longevity through the lens of health and well-being.

Each chapter begins with a well-known quote to introduce the reader to an overview of a self-care strategy. This is an excellent way to capture the reader's attention and begin their self-reflection while providing them with a short glimpse of what they can expect to discover throughout the chapter. Most superintendents often view their work through the lens of their current realities, educational trends, and small life events.

Prioritizing Health and Well-Being provides readers with a descriptor to ponder as they begin to explore the possibilities of self-care in each chapter to address the current realities. Each chapter is formatted the same to help organize the information in a practical and easy-to-use format for the reader. The descriptor (or quote) provides the reader with a glimpse of what each chapter is about.

The body (or introduction) of each chapter provides the overarching importance of the self-care principle or topic for each chapter. The principle, strategy, or topic is presented in words and supported through practical terms, which explains why self-care is critical to the overall effectiveness and health of superintendents. The Practical Strategies section is often a favorite section for readers, as it provides strategies focused on a healthy work-life balance—in other words, how superintendents can apply the strategy to their own lives.

The practical strategies section is critical for several reasons: 1) Through experience, I am familiar with each strategy to offer advice to aspiring, novice, or veteran superintendents. 2) I believe it is essential for each reader to have quick access to strategies that are practical and can be quickly adopted and utilized. 3) The strategies are presented in simple terms, as they are easy to use.

The Voices from the Field section provides the reader with a short example of each self-care principle presented through the perspective of a practitioner (a current or former superintendent). The reader is given a glimpse of leadership self-care through the lens of short stories, a type of case study of a leadership moment. The best way to gain an understanding of each self-care principle is to see how superintendents have transformed their superintendency through a focus on self-care.

In the examples provided, the superintendent can begin to or continue their focus on their health or well-being, to extend their longevity as a leader, find a healthier work-life balance, and improve their overall effectiveness as the chief executive officer of a school district. The Key Takeaway section serves as a summary of the chapter in simple form so that they can quickly review the principles, strategies, and topics covered in the chapter.

Prepare yourself for a journey that will help you improve your effectiveness as a superintendent, through a focus on your health and well-being.

CHAPTER ONE

The Transformative Three

"We never know the worth of water till the well is dry."
—French Proverb

In education, transformation is often loosely used by educators, school administrators, and superintendents. Typically, transformation is focused on something in education, such as school transformation, instructional transformation, culture transformation, and the list goes on. But in this case, transformation is focused on the rejuvenation of the mind, body, and spirit. Yes, there needs to be a transformation within the superintendency focused on the health and well-being of superintendents.

Superintendents can transform their leadership, health, and well-being by drinking water, ensuring they get enough sleep, and exercising at least four days a week. All three are free but are often elusive to most superintendents. The superintendency is hard and getting more complicated with each passing day. As such, superintendents are prone to let their health and well-being fall by the wayside as they go full steam ahead in their jobs.

In the back of a superintendent's mind is the recognition that going full speed without breaks or focusing on their health is a recipe for disaster, yet too many plow ahead with full force. When leaders only focus on bottom-line numbers (performance), their own well-being and the well-being of students, teachers, and staff are often neglected. Though well-being is seldom discussed in superintendent preparation programs or in research, it is not something to overlook.

Though water, sleep, and exercise are available to all superintendents, few recognize the benefits that each one brings to their leadership and overall health and well-being. Go into any superintendent's office and more than likely you will see coffee mugs or soda cans, with a few water bottles hidden behind soda or energy drinks. Superintendents who drink coffee and soda will tell you that they need caffeine, but all they are doing is disguising other severe issues such as a lack of exercise, energy, and sleep. Some drink coffee or soda all throughout the day, just to make it through the workday with periods of drops in energy as the caffeine and sugar wear off.

Water is transformative because it not only helps to break the addiction to caffeine and sugar but also replenishes our bodies and minds. Though breaking the addiction to caffeine can be a lengthy process for many, once water is the drink of choice, transformation begins. Superintendents will have more energy throughout the day without periods of drops of energy, sleep better, and feel like they have clearer thoughts. Eight to ten glasses of water are all a person needs each day, and with each sip of water the superintendent will become more effective in their jobs.

Though water is important, sleep is the next most important strategy in the superintendent's journey to rejuvenate their health and well-being, as well as their leadership. Most superintendents will attest that they get extraordinarily little sleep through the week, going to bed late and getting up early. Most adults need between six to eight hours of sleep to function effectively, but few ever reach that, settling for four to five hours of sleep.

A lack of sleep is dangerous over the long term. It can lead to obesity, heart issues, hormonal issues, accelerated aging, a weakened immune system, and the list continues. Overall, a lack of sleep negatively impacts our health and well-being, which then prevents superintendents from being effective leaders. Superintendents think they can function on little sleep, but in reality they are impacting their health, as well as their careers, for the long term.

Superintendents never turn themselves off—at night, over the weekend, or even on vacation. When most superintendents lay down at night to sleep, their minds keep going, thinking about a decision that has been made, tomorrow's schedule, or the pressures of the job. No wonder many can't get proper amounts of sleep. Superintendents must get to a point of stopping making excuses for not being able to sleep at night and finding solutions and strategies to get the recommended amount of sleep that they need.

The last of the three is exercise. Just like water and sleep, too many superintendents have not made their schedules accommodating of exercise. Superintendents' schedules are insanely packed each day, starting early in the morning and going late into the night as they meet with community members, board members, or attend school performances or athletic events. As they try to squeeze so much into their daily schedules, they are rarely available for their health, much less exercise.

This is not to say that there are not superintendents who have unlocked secrets to exercise, but most superintendents have not exercised in years, and it is often noticeable both at work and at home. Plagued by ongoing fatigue, loss of energy, obesity, and many other things, superintendents who fail to exercise daily struggle each day. The thing to keep in mind is that exercise, something as simple as walking, is foreign to too many superintendents.

Most superintendents, like most Americans, are overweight, have an unhealthy diet, and exercise little, with some not exercising at all. When leaders exercise, they experience lower levels of stress, have better health overall, and lead more effectively. Exercise allows superintendents to work out their stress and helps to clarify their thoughts and decisions. Exercise is truly an amazing strategy to better health and leadership, and it goes unknown to far too many superintendents.

Regular exercise, finding twenty minutes to forty-five minutes each day, can be transformative to a superintendent's life and leadership. Exercise can be as simple as walking outside, walking on a treadmill at a school's gym, or walking around the gym floor. Exercise does not require an expensive gym membership; that is only another excuse that many superintendents develop that prevents them from realizing the power of exercise in their lives and leadership. Exercise is discussed more in-depth later in chapter 20.

Of all the chapters in this book, this chapter is the most important, because it is the most transformative and commonsensical. Sadly, all three, water, sleep, and exercise are available to everyone for free, yet are elusive to so many superintendents due to obstacles that the superintendency has created. These constructs are man-made and can be removed by each superintendent if they choose to make their health and well-being a priority in their lives and leadership. Try all three—become addicted to all three, and watch how your health, well-being, and leadership improve overnight.

Practical Strategies

1. *Start small.* Too many superintendents will attempt to go cold turkey with sodas or whatever their drink of choice, or to try to sleep more, or to go and purchase expensive gym memberships or buy television-inspired exercise programs. As a leader, you are encouraged to take each day as a step closer to drinking more water, getting more sleep,

and exercising each day. Gradual progress is better for the long term and helps you to become acclimated to the changes.

2. *Recognize and remove.* Pick a day of the week and evaluate what you drink, eat, how many hours of sleep you get, how much you exercise or move, and what makes up most of your schedule. Before one can change, one must first recognize that you have a problem and then develop a plan to move forward. It will shock most superintendents about what they do each day without even thinking about it. Likewise, most superintendents will be shocked by what they drink, eat, what clogs up your schedule, and what they do just before bed. To start the path to wellness, you must first admit that you have a problem with your own health and well-being.

3. *Schedule priorities.* Superintendents must carve out time each day dedicated to their health and well-being, no matter if they schedule their own appointments or if they have an assistant that does their schedule for them. Superintendents need time to themselves to disconnect, breathe, and, yes, exercise. Again, this can be simply walking outside on a treadmill, around the gym, or performing school-building walkthroughs. Just move—that is what is most important. Sitting behind your desk all day is detrimental to your health, and there is nothing that speeds up aging than staying sedentary for prolonged periods of the day. The superintendency, if you're not careful, can confine a leader behind the desk. They must resist this temptation and exercise as much as they can to counteract job-related tendencies.

Voices from the Field

Water . . . Does the Body Good

Dr. Ed Smith is a fifty-nine-year-old male, who has been a superintendent of a rural school district in the southeast with 1,500 students for fifteen years. He didn't realize how little water he drank each day. One day he decided to pay attention to exactly what he drank and was shocked. He realized that the only time he was drinking water, less than a glass, was each morning when he took his prescriptions for high blood pressure and cholesterol.

He was drinking eight cups of coffee in the morning and immediately switching to a diet soda about 10:00 a.m. and continuing every two hours, like clockwork. He could easily drink six to nine cans of soda by 5:00 p.m. each day. When he got home, he would drink whatever was in the refrigerator, which did little for his health. At ball games, he would have more soft drinks, when he could easily have chosen water but opted for the soft drink.

After visiting his physician one day for a regular check-up, he finally decided that he would start cutting back on the soda. His physician was concerned about the level of sugar based on his recent labs and for his age. He thought to himself that he was drinking himself to death—not with alcohol but with soda drinks. As he was heading back to the office from his doctor's appointment he went by the supermarket and picked up a forty-eight pack of water bottles, and he slowly started cutting back on sodas.

Dr. Smith started slowly cutting back each day to give his body an opportunity to acclimate to the drop in sugar and caffeine. He had been drinking so much coffee and soda for so long, he knew if he didn't start slow, he would crash and immediately return to his habit of drinking coffee and soda all day long. He admits he still drinks soft drinks, but he only has one with his lunch and at dinner.

Ed now averages between six to eight bottles of water each day, and overall, he feels better. At first, he struggled as he thought he would, but he just kept telling himself it would get easier tomorrow. When he visited his physician a couple of months later, he told him he felt so much better that he couldn't imagine going back to his reliance on coffee and sodas. This year marks year eight of making the switch to water.

Dr. Smith feels so much better and has more energy than he did when I started serving as a superintendent. His overall health has improved, he lost about twenty-five pounds, and his blood pressure is stable. He will admit he didn't just drink water to lose weight but also started walking daily. Still, he looks at each day as a new opportunity to make progress. If he had made the change before he did, I wonder where he would be, personally and professionally. But he is so proud of his progress and self-accountability.

Key Takeaway

There are so many forces that are in play that could derail a superintendent—including their own health. The simplest way for a superintendent to take back their health is to drink water, sleep, and exercise. The "three" are freely available to every superintendent across the nation, yet few recognize or take advantage of them. You must not allow excuses to keep you from focusing on your own health and well-being. Some good advice is for superintendents to fill the refrigerator at their offices with water or to purchase filtered water fountains, make it a priority to get to bed early and disconnect from work, and schedule time for exercise each day. Super-intendents can control so much in their personal and professional lives—if they choose to.

CHAPTER TWO

The Sun Will Rise Tomorrow

"Even the darkest night will end, and the sun will rise again."
—Victor Hugo

Each day brings a new opportunity. There are days as a superintendent when many are left to wonder if the next day will be an improvement or a continuation of the same stress, roadblocks, stumbles, mistakes, and other obstacles. The longer a person remains as superintendent, the more they will see days that they wish had never occurred—it's inevitable. There will undoubtedly be days and weeks that are tough, but superintendents must keep moving forward, holding fast to their purpose, values, and vision, and know that tomorrow will certainly be better than today.

Superintendents, like others, must believe that the sun will in fact rise tomorrow. Leaders without hope lead to employees without hope and an organization rudderless in a changing and dynamic sea. When superintendents lose hope of tomorrow, they begin to blame themselves for whatever has transpired and experience fatigue, exhaustion, and other health ailments. Depression is much more than a case of the blues; it can be long-term and debilitating to so many adults in America.

Countless leaders, including superintendents, experience depression from work-related factors, and in most cases, it stems from the lack of confidence in themselves and a hope for a better tomorrow. There are times when superintendents get so down on themselves, they can't possibly be mentally prepared to lead. Furthermore, if superintendents are not careful, the job can become so overwhelming that many begin to contemplate resigning or retiring. The superintendency is not for the faint of heart.

As superintendents grow older the risk of depression and feelings of hopelessness increase because of changes in their moods, hormones, and body. What may have been a simple chore five years ago is now a daunting task today. What may have been easy decisions yesterday prove to be harder today. Plus, every morning as superintendents stare into the mirror, they see firsthand how the job has aged them, sometimes overnight.

As such, many say to themselves that they can't go on, they can't do the job any longer, or they ask themselves why they have worked tirelessly only to look like they do—gray, wrinkles, slumping body posture, increasing weight, or all of the above and then some. This could be hard for even the most seasoned and self-confident superintendent. The superintendency, when not kept in balance, has a negative impact on a person's health and well-being, and their work-life balance.

Obviously, most superintendents focus on external appearance and regularly forget about their inner health. Though the superintendent may have aged, tomorrow can be bright. Age and hope can coexist. Superintendents must look at tomorrow as an opportunity to improve, grow, and change the trajectory for themselves, their school district, and, more importantly, their students. No matter how bad today might be, tomorrow always begins with a clean slate, whether righting the wrongs of yesterday or charting a new journey for the future.

Superintendents can't allow a single day or week to determine their careers. The only thing each day requires is that they give the job 100 percent of their effort, dedication, and heart. Though some days will be harder than others, at the end of the day, superintendents can only give what they have, no more and no less. The number of bad days pale in comparison to the many good days superintendents will experience over the course of their superintendency. Though on the worst day, many may have questioned their own leadership, why it was happening to them, and how they are going to move forward, they are still a superintendent.

To maintain their health and well-being and remain effective as a leader, superintendents must believe that tomorrow will always be better. This isn't encouraging a superintendent to live in la-la land but to develop the mental and physical stamina to believe in tomorrow, no matter how bad today may get. It's not emotionally, mentally, or physically healthy to not believe that tomorrow will be better. The belief that the sun will rise tomorrow is a powerful, transformational, and rejuvenating force personally and professionally. Furthermore, the hope of tomorrow is a calming force on those days that are trying and stressing to a superintendent's health and well-being.

Practical Strategies

1. *Recognize all the positives.* There are so many positives that happen each day, but superintendents often focus only on the negatives. Negativity is contagious, and if leaders are negative then the entire organizational culture is negative. Though remaining positive may be hard on particularly stressful days, you must always celebrate and recognize the many positives that happen in your life and in the job. Though this may be hard for many superintendents, especially with the number of decisions they make and the number of interactions they have each day, the positives exist and should outweigh the negatives.

2. *Reflect on the positives.* If the positives are outnumbered by negatives each day, create more positives. Superintendents must create more positive outcomes in the office or in schools. They must schedule positive things on their calendars so that it forces them to have a brighter day and hope for tomorrow. They must make it a goal to get out of their offices as much as possible, as headaches have an easy path to find them when they are shackled behind a desk. Problems and trouble can find them if they are fixed to their chairs—as most seasoned superintendents have discovered.

3. *Multitask within limits.* When things begin to pile up on a superintendent's desk, they become overwhelmed and their mood changes—it's natural. Instead of trying to be everywhere at one time and always involved in every decision, they must try to focus on one task at a time, giving their attention to priorities, allowing themselves to relish the positives of the experience. When they multitask or overextend themselves each day, as leaders, they can't experience the positives of the job, as they try to get to the next task at hand.

Voices from the Field

The Healing Power of the Sunrise

Patricia Allen is a forty-seven-year-old superintendent of a suburban school district who has served for three years, serving 5400 students in the Midwest. When she started out as a superintendent, each day was like drinking water from a fire hydrant with a steady, pressurized stream of water. Before she got into her vehicle to drive to work each day, she was already answering phone calls or replying to emails or texts. Patricia's schedule was jam-packed each day from sunrise to well past sunset. Her first two years were like this with few breaks.

Mrs. Allen got to the point that all she thought about was the job, and she sadly recounts how being a wife and mother was a distant second. She got caught in the cycle of the superintendency that demanded all her attention each day. Regretfully, she missed family get-togethers, worked on vacations, and even checked text messages during church services. The job was consuming her life.

Her work schedule got so bad that if she wasn't working, she felt out of place. As the job became normal, life became a second priority. She was drowning, and she couldn't stop. One evening she was working late at the office, and she began to cry because she knew that the next day was going to be just like the day before—no breaks, back-to-back meetings, arriving home well after dinner with her family. For the first time, she felt depressed and helpless. She wanted to call the board chair and tell him she was resigning immediately.

Mrs. Allen became a victim of the job, and she swore she would never be a victim of anything or anyone. The proverbial line in the sand was staring at her, and she knew she had to make a change. Instead of dreading tomorrow, Patricia should have been looking at tomorrow as a renewal opportunity to recommit to what matters most to her. Late that evening, she pushed the paperwork and emails to the side of her desk and started looking at how she could change tomorrow.

Instead of being confined to meetings, she wanted her day filled with school experiences, interacting with students, teachers, custodians, bus drivers—the people who really need her. But also, she wanted to be home in time for dinner with her family, which she knew was going to be hard, but doable. She wanted to hear about her kids' day at school and help them with homework, an opportunity to be a mother that had been placed on hold for far too long.

That night she finally decided to change the narrative. Patricia was no longer going to allow the job to control her happiness. She was no longer going to become stressed and depressed about tomorrow but excited about the opportunity to make it positive for herself, her family, and her students and staff. In many respects, she is happy that the pressures of the job got to her early, as she knew other superintendents spend their entire careers unhappy, controlled by the job, as they lose everything that is important to them.

Sometimes unhappiness must occur before someone can truly cherish happiness. Now, Patricia is in her third year as superintendent, and each day, she goes to bed at night blessed with happiness and hope. Mrs. Allen hopes that others will find hope and happiness. It's there, if superintendents will search for it. It's not that hard, but superintendents must first recognize that they don't need to give up everything in their life for the sake of the job.

Key Takeaway

No one is guaranteed tomorrow, but that doesn't mean that superintendents can't look at the opportunities that tomorrow will bring. Though superintendents are facing an unprecedented climate and attitudes toward public education today, there are still more positives than negatives. Though difficult, this is precisely the moment when superintendents must focus on a better and brighter tomorrow. Each day, superintendents must convey hope as much as possible, while also being a realist. In times of crisis or change, stakeholders look to the superintendent, you, to provide transparency, empathy, stability, and hope for a better tomorrow. Though it may be painful and tough today, you must describe the path forward.

The pressure for superintendents to be leaders of hope of tomorrow is a daunting task, especially when there are so many things happening in public education today. But the more you, as the leader, practice hope, the easier it becomes each day. Hope doesn't come naturally for some leaders, but this is what they need and what their followers need. Superintendents will be surprised by how transformative hope can be on their health, effectiveness, and their organization. If you focus on the positives and believe that tomorrow will be better, you will have more energy, feel better, and overall experience better health—ultimately, you will be less exhausted.

CHAPTER THREE

Be Comfortable in Your Own Skin

"To be yourself in a world that is constantly trying to make you something else is the greatest accomplishment."

—Ralph Waldo Emerson

Educators want to become superintendents because they believe they can lead the educational system. They feel that they possess the talents, skills, characteristics, personality, and mindset to lead effectively. Every new superintendent starts out with a burst of energy, a sense of renewed commitment to lead and learn. Over time, though, something changes along the way for many superintendents—where the energy dissipates, the passion for the work fizzles, and their health isn't quite what it used to be.

The story sounds too familiar in today's school districts. Superintendents begin to become leaders they are not or try to disguise who they really are. Each leader is uniquely wired to lead in a certain way. When they try to change and be someone they are not, the damage to their emotional, mental, and physical health and overall well-being is impacted greatly. If you look at pictures of superintendents in their first year and then three or four years later, their image is starkly different.

Superintendents stare in wonder of what happened and then conclude the job got the best of the person in the picture—usually, they are looking at their own photo. The person's photo shows an individual who is tired, mentally exhausted by the look in their eyes, a little chubbier in the cheeks due to a poor diet, dark and heavy bags under their eyes, and a little lighter in the hair due to graying. The transformation is astonishing . . . in a bad way.

Superintendents who are comfortable with who they are fair so much better than those who try to be a leader they are not. It's hard to stay true to yourself in a very dynamic and changing work environment such as education. Education remains in flux, especially over the past decade. Pressures of the educational system force superintendents into a path that many are not accustomed to. Some do well with change, but most superintendents are not comfortable with it and develop stress-related apathy toward the job and the bureaucracy, which begins to chip away at their well-being.

Pretending to be someone they are not results in burnout, unnecessary stress, and feelings of dislike toward oneself. The superintendency naturally comes with stress—that's the job. Superintendents are responsible for the safety of students and employees and the level of learning by students. Those are two major responsibilities that undoubtedly are stressful. Superintendents don't need to exacerbate their stress levels by trying to lead in a way that is misaligned with their talents or skills. This only leads to higher levels of stress, which impact the leader's overall health and well-being.

Before accepting the superintendent's job, the leader must really do their homework to ensure their leadership style, skills, and talents are aligned with what the district needs and the board of education demands. No one can mask their leadership for long; either their true self comes out or they burn out and leave, or both. The diversity of need for superintendents is as great as the number of districts that have vacancies each year for their chief executive officer. Instead of rushing to find a job, any job, the superintendent, for the sake of their own health, must give their due diligence in ensuring the talent set is aligned to the needs of the job.

Understandably, districts change over time—which may require a different skillset from a superintendent. This is where the superintendent must have confidence in their leadership skills and either be steadfast with their own style or leave, but never compromise their own style to conform to the need and situation. It does not work and never ends with positive results for the district or the superintendent, professionally or personally.

Practical Strategies

1. *Fully understand who the board of education is seeking.* What kind of leader does the district need? What are the superintendent's goals, skills, and talents? Superintendents must not rush to get a job and pretend to be someone they are not. This never works and can cause long-term damage to your health, well-being, and career.

2. *Be honest with yourself.* Superintendents must walk comfortably in their own shoes each day. They must not hide who they are. Though they may have to be willing to relocate, there is a superintendency that needs their particular skills and talents. Settling for the first job offer may prove to be a mistake for them professionally and personally. Misalignment between their skills and style and the job will lead to unbearable stress.

3. *Be comfortable with your style.* Superintendents who hide who they are, over time, will gradually have long-term health conditions. Hiding behind a facade will only lead the superintendent so far, but when it is removed the long-term impact is much greater than if they were honest from the start. Boards of education want superintendents who are comfortable with their own leadership styles and willing to lead. Boards of education want them to be successful and that begins first with making sure you know who you are as a leader.

Voices from the Field

Learn the Hard Way

Miguel Johnson is a fifty-five-year-old male, who has been a superintendent of an urban school district located in the southeast. Miguel has been a superintendent for ten years—five years in a previous school district, and now in his fifth year in his current school district. During his first tenure as superintendent, having served as a principal and then a district administrator in the same school district was not as rewarding as his current position.

He had a good relationship with his board and knew what they expected of him, but he couldn't be who they needed him to be. They weren't asking him to do anything illegal or unethical but things that simply did not align with his overall goals, values, and principles. When he interviewed for the previous position as superintendent, he had been in the district for several years, serving in multiple roles.

Mr. Johnson knew precisely what the board expected from the superintendent. He had many of the board members' kids in school as their principal, so he had several firsthand experiences and interactions with them that allowed him to understand who they were looking for when hiring a superintendent. After serving at the district level for three years, the superintendent position came available when the previous superintendent announced his retirement. He and the former superintendent were completely different; he was effective, but they had different leadership styles.

Miguel had been through superintendent preparation programs offered by his state association and had the credentials to be a superintendent. In his mind, he was prepared, and he knew what at least five of the seven board members were looking for in a superintendent. He was prepared extensively for the interview like every other applicant. He knew he wasn't a sure winner for the position, but he had a better than fifty-fifty chance of getting hired. He was hired unanimously by the board, which helped him to start strong.

From day one, Miguel quickly realized he was in over his head, not on policy matters or leadership decisions, but in the way that his beliefs and the direction of the board were misaligned. Within months he was already feeling stressed and each day he felt like he was experiencing a severe panic attack. Prior to the superintendency, he had never experienced anything close to a panic attack. He cringed every time he met with a board member, and he felt nauseous prior to each monthly board meeting. Miguel started vomiting before each board meeting due to nerves, and during board meetings he would freeze—he couldn't speak or advise the board effectively.

Mr. Johnson's health condition was all because when he interviewed, he pretended to be someone he was not, and when he got the position, he tried to be something the board didn't need, but who he was. The board was professional about their concerns with his leadership, never broadcasting their concerns publicly, and he appreciated that, but he still knew if he stayed in the position for the long term, he would eventually experience more severe health issues. He went to his physician, and he was told that the best prescription was to let go of the job because no medication was going to solve his health problems.

Sadly, Miguel learned the hard way that he had to be comfortable in his own skin and that pretending to be a leader he was not was detrimental to his health. He knew better, but he had to learn the hard way. He was one of the lucky ones, as his body was telling him early on that he could not keep pretending. Unfortunately, he knew that many others try to push through and weather on, only to find out too late they pretended too long. He now tells aspiring superintendents to be comfortable with who they are. Don't change just to get a job, as there are school districts that are looking for their talents and skills.

Key Takeaway

The superintendency only gets more dynamic and more difficult with each passing day. Superintendents must be comfortable in their own shoes and skin. Trying to be something they are not results in destroyed careers, burnout, exhaustion, and long-term health issues. Those superintendents who are not afraid to be themselves and who are proud of their skills, talents, and experiences are far more likely to remain in the job than those who pretend to be something they are not.

Imagine the weight of the stress of those superintendents who work in a superintendency with a misalignment between their style and the needs of the organization. Each day worried that their true selves will be revealed. It happens far too often and damages careers, school districts, and an individual's health and well-being. Superintendents must be principled in their resolve to be who they are as leaders and members of a team. They can only be themselves if they expect to be successful.

Superintendents must never compromise their leadership style and principles. High-performing superintendents are confident of their abilities and understand the importance of the alignment between their talents and the job. The longevity of superintendents is dependent on so many factors, including a leader's health. Superintendents who find themselves in a situation where there is a misalignment between their talents, skills, and style with the demands of the job are destined for a noticeably short tenure in the office.

Just as a person who is not a marathon runner shouldn't register for and run in the Boston Marathon, a superintendent who doesn't possess the skill set of a particular superintendency should not accept the job. Both the person who isn't trained to run a marathon and the person who doesn't have the skills and talents for the superintendency will experience long-term health conditions that may not only end a career but also result in significant injury to their health and well-being. You can do permanent damage to your health, well-being, and career if you're not honest and comfortable with yourself personally and professionally.

CHAPTER FOUR

Put Your Oxygen Mask on Before Helping Others

"Whenever you feel compelled to put others first at the expense of yourself, you are denying your own reality, your own identity."

—David Stafford

If you have flown lately or over the past decade, right before takeoff, the flight attendant will remind everyone that in the event of an emergency, oxygen masks will drop from the ceiling and to please place your oxygen mask on before helping someone else. Superintendents are trained to take care of others before focusing on themselves. This is an excellent leadership trait that leaders take; however, when it comes to health and well-being, superintendents need to first focus on their own health before helping others.

There are so many examples of superintendents prioritizing health, well-being, and success before themselves. It comes with the job. Leaders take all the criticism but share any success with others. This self-sacrificing mentality is admirable and commendable. There can never be enough true leaders who lead because they want the responsibility of leading transformation, serving others, and creating positive outcomes for students. There is a growing number of leaders, including superintendents, who want the title but not the responsibility, so how do we fault those who are willing to go the extra mile even at the cost of their own health and well-being?

Most will celebrate the work ethic and leadership of superintendents who lead through service, but all that is happening is that we are adding to the increasing superintendent burnout by applauding long hours.

Superintendents, like other educators, are working themselves to death, and with extraordinarily little to show for it. They get lost in the job and forget about one of the most important things—their own health and well-being.

Students, teachers, staff members, parents, guardians, and the community need superintendents that desire to have longevity in the job. Working around the clock, eating poorly, not exercising, or not taking any time away from the job does not equate to longevity in any organization, especially schools. Make no mistake, being an educator or superintendent in today's schools is extremely difficult.

The demands are crippling on multiple levels, which is why the average tenure of a superintendent is three to five years. But what is alarming is that that number continues to decrease as the pressures continue to mount with each passing year. Since the beginning of the COVID-19 pandemic, the turnover rate and burnout have only increased, and the forecast for the superintendency does not appear to be promising for the next several years.

At some point in time, superintendents must make their health their number one priority if they expect to have a chance at longevity and any level of success. Though success can be measured in a variety of ways, their overall health is typically not a metric that is discussed. Superintendents should have annual exams with their local physician or one that specializes in preventive care. It is perfectly acceptable for a superintendent to focus on their health. In fact, most boards of education would contend that if the superintendent isn't healthy, then the district isn't healthy.

With everything going on in education today, and as schools continue to navigate all the complexities associated with COVID-19, now is a perfect time to focus on the health and well-being of superintendents. There is no shame in acknowledging that something about the job must change if the expectation is a long tenure as a superintendent. The days of eighty-hour workweeks, constantly checking email, texts, and social media posts, and no separation between work and life are gone.

Today's superintendents need to lead, work effectively and efficiently, prioritize their health and well-being, and model the way for others. These four things, if adopted, can prove to be transformative for any superintendent. You can be an effective superintendent if you first make your own health the priority. Realize that boards of education, teachers, staff, and students need you to be healthy and in a good place with your own well-being. If you struggle, they too will struggle.

Practical Strategies

1. *Schedule time for yourself.* Finding at least twenty minutes each day to read, walk, listen to music, breathe, or just sit in silence, can rejuvenate your health and well-being. Superintendents have a certain level of control over their schedule and prioritize what matters to them. Their health and well-being should always be at the top of their priority list. Scheduling time for themselves does not impede their ability to do their jobs and serve others, but in fact, strengthens their ability to be effective.

2. *Exercise the no option.* The quantity of items on a calendar does not equate to effectiveness as a superintendent but will certainly lead to exhaustion and burnout. Superintendents cannot do everything within a twenty-four-hour window, and they are not expected to be able to do so. Their health and well-being, as leaders, are placed under elevated levels of stress when they overextend themselves. Less is more—say no and delegate. Know your limits and don't be afraid to say you need a break or delegate to others. You are not shifting responsibility, but instead, making sure you can be effective and healthy!

3. *Check your balance.* Before superintendents take on someone else's burden, they must make sure that they first make sure that they are balanced and okay. Taking on additional burdens before getting themselves in check never helps anyone. Superintendents rarely, due to time and other priorities, check themselves, specifically their health and well-being. When their health and well-being are not in a good place, they are not leading but only surviving. They cannot effectively help others with their health and well-being, if their life, work, and health are out of balance.

4. *Use the brake pad.* Superintendents must start listening to what their bodies are telling them. Everyone's, not just superintendents', bodies have an early warning system that will alert them if they are approaching exhaustion and burnout. Bodies will begin to shut down out of protection. Recognizing your limits, knowing when to slow down change, and changing the course before it's too late can save your health and well-being. If you are constantly getting home from work at the breaking point, stop, reflect, and make a change in your trajectory quickly. It is easy to work yourself to a point of no return.

Voices from the Field

The Leader's Health First, A New Concept

Richard Lincoln is a fifty-one-year-old male who has been a superintendent of a rural school district in the northwest for ten years. He considers himself a healthy superintendent. He has always made his health a priority, going all the way back to college. He has always been an avid runner, trying to run at least ten miles per week, while also going to the gym at least three to four times each week.

His health is important, not just professionally, but also personally. When he became superintendent, his world was turned upside down. He quickly realized that his workout and running schedule was not meshing with his professional calendar as a superintendent. He remembers that during his first six months he may have gone to the gym three times. Compare that to his workout routine prior to becoming a superintendent, and obviously there is a significant difference.

After the first couple of months, Mr. Lincoln could notice a difference in his body. His joints started to ache, his sleep pattern changed, and he found himself eating more, which is abnormal for him. He was "stress" eating—which isn't good for anyone, no matter how healthy the person may be. In the first six months, he gained at least ten pounds. His body was transforming in front of him, and it was all because of the job.

When he became superintendent, he put his health on hold because of the demands of the job. Richard was so focused on the job that even though he felt different, he didn't know how to put the brakes on. He started the superintendency on July 1, and by December of that year, the job had taken a toll on his health, marriage, and his effectiveness as a leader. As he prioritized the job, he let things that were important to him be put on the back-burner, including his marriage.

Luckily, his wife gave him a lot of latitude; she understood what he was going through. Many superintendent's marriages end because of the demands of the job. She had a lot of patience as they stopped going out on the weekends and taking road trips because he was always at the office or attending an extracurricular event or community meeting. She was worried about his health but was reluctant to say anything, though she would ask if he went to the gym.

Even for a superintendent that had prioritized his health all his life, the job got the best of Mr. Lincoln. Just imagine what happens to a superintendent who has never made their health a priority. To him, he was not leading effectively. He was jumping from one fire to another every day, going from meeting to meeting, without ever giving himself a break. He wasn't helping anyone, including himself.

He was burned out, and he was only six months into the job. That January, right after winter recess for the school district, he scheduled a time to speak with the chair and vice chair of the board of education. All through the winter recess he was nervous, and he didn't really want to talk to the board about his health. Surprisingly, the meeting went well, and he didn't expect the outcome.

Both the board chair and vice chair, who are professionals in the community, told Mr. Lincoln that he had to make his health a priority, because if not, he wouldn't be around for long. They encouraged him to delegate more and find time for his health and marriage. They explained to him one of the reasons that they hired him was because they knew he was healthy and hopefully would be in the district a while, as the three previous superintendents were at the end of their careers and only stayed two or three years each. They wanted a superintendent with longevity to stabilize the district, and his health was a major factor in doing so.

The district, specifically the board, needed Mr. Lincoln to prioritize his health so that he could help others. He was not doing anyone any favors by allowing the job to consume his life. His health was important to him and to his ability to lead effectively, and he needed to return to focusing on his health. It wasn't easy, but he realized that he had to do something. Over the next four to five months, he paid attention to his health, prioritized his schedule, and spent time with his wife whenever he could.

Mr. Lincoln realizes that he is fortunate to have a board that understood the importance of his health, as many do not. After he got his schedule back in balance, he began scheduling regular time for running and the gym, and time with his wife through the week and on weekends. He credits the board chair and vice chair for stepping up, focusing on his health, and giving him permission to "put his oxygen mask on first."

Key Takeaway

It may seem like a broken record that plays repeatedly but prioritizing your health through a daily schedule is key. Superintendents become so busy and focus on the health and well-being of others, they forget about their own health and well-being. Superintendents who do not focus on their health are not leading but only surviving. Too many superintendents crawl into work each day, trying to help others, when in fact, they have every opportunity to put their health and well-being first.

Over the past several decades, leaders, including superintendents, have placed value on the well-being of others, while their own health and well-being have become elusive. People ask, "Why are so many superintendents leaving the profession?" and the answer is clear—burnout, exhaustion, stress, and an unhealthy work-life balance. Leadership must be sustainable in an organization. Sustainability requires a healthy leader and healthy organizational culture. Public education today needs healthy leaders who can lead without compromising their own health, which has been the standard for too long. To truly make student and teacher well-being a priority, you, as the leader, must make your well-being a priority first.

CHAPTER FIVE

Use the Chisel

"Don't accept the limitations of other people who claim things are 'unchangeable.' If it's written in stone, bring your hammer and chisel."
—Peter McWilliams

Superintendents are ridiculously hard on themselves. Too many superintendents take everything personally—whether that is student test scores, teacher turnover, budget deficits, community support, and so on. With every component of the school district, superintendents struggle to let go and to not take things personally. Some will argue that leaders must take things personally if they are to be effective. That may be true but not to the point it destroys their career and health.

Each day, superintendents must chisel away things that they think make them ineffective. Superintendents are humans just like everyone else, but at the end of the day, they must be able to bear the burdens of the district. As a result, superintendents take on and carry a lot of personal and organizational baggage that eventually consumes them. Humans can only take so much before exhaustion sets in, and too many superintendents are approaching extraneous exhaustion that is bad not only for the organization but also for their leadership and overall health.

Superintendents, hopefully sooner rather than later, must be willing to reflect and pick up the tool and start chiseling away at the pressures, stress, burdens, and everything else that may come with the job. This is not to say that superintendents should throw up their hands and give up or become less accessible or visible in the district. Chiseling away the stress is about prioritizing components of the job that are most important to the organization, as well as the superintendent on a personal and professional level.

With every stroke of the hammer against the chisel head, the superintendent frees up time, space, and burdens. Chiseling is transformative to leaders. It is both a professional and personal process, whereby the superintendent becomes more effective as a leader, regains their health, and becomes more present and connected with themselves and their families. Longevity as a superintendent requires the leader to chisel often and make sure that they have prioritized the most important things in life.

Chiseling is the process of prioritizing what matters most to them, personally and professionally. It is an exceedingly arduous process for superintendents, as they are involved in so many things each day, and most job descriptions are lengthy and, in some cases, ridiculously too rigid. From board relations, budgets, and community outreach to student achievement and attendance, the superintendent plays a key role in the district.

Chiseling requires the superintendent to drill down to what matters most, to schedule accordingly, and to maximize opportunities to focus on their own health and well-being. Superintendents must become more aware of themselves, their jobs, and the unintended consequences of carrying extra baggage. Just as a constant drip of water from a leaky faucet can fill a sink over time, the constant drip of stress, pressure, burdens, and around-the-clock work hours, will eventually negatively impact the superintendent's health and even their professional career. Time always catches up with leaders!

Let's be real, leaders may think that working around the clock is a good standard to set in the organization, but it does the opposite. Employees want leaders who will be there for the long haul. This requires a superintendent who understands and values their own health and well-being. When employees see leaders burning the midnight oil and taking no time off, they begin to disengage from work because they are afraid that they are not living up to the impossible expectations of prioritizing work over their own well-being.

Taking time each week to chisel away things that are not required personally and professionally will go a long way in prioritizing a superintendent's life. Superintendents have an awesome opportunity to change the course of the history of the district, especially student learning and teacher development, but if they are bogged down in nonprioritized things, their impact is lessened. The goal is to make sure that superintendents have a lengthy career, and that can only happen by prioritizing their leadership and well-being.

Practical Strategies

1. *Realize that change is possible.* The superintendency is dynamic and complicated. Superintendents often lead within confines that have developed over decades. This doesn't mean that change can't happen. Superintendents must initiate change across the district and even in their own position. You, in your role as a leader, must identify what needs to change and work to make the change happen—personally and professionally. If you don't make change happen, then change will not happen, especially when it comes to your health and well-being.

2. *Recognize limits.* Every leader has limits, including superintendents. Some superintendents will be able to multitask better than others. Each superintendent will need to know their limits in what they can handle at one time. Adding more things to their plate that they can't handle will only lead to stress, anxiety, feelings of loss of control, and other health issues. You must manage your workload. Once you reach your limit, and you know your limit, stop taking on the stresses, pressures, and burdens of everyone else. You can only handle so much as the leader and remain effective and . . . healthy!

3. *Unload and release.* If superintendents are carrying a lot, they must start chiseling away the things that are not on their priority list, personally and professionally. There are only so many hours in a day, and no one can work around the clock and expect to be healthy, effective, and have longevity in their position. Not everything is a priority, and you must decide what must be prioritized based on your overall health and well-being. You must find strategies that help you with stress relief, but first, you must start with those tangible things in your life that may lead to stress and an unhealthy work-life balance.

4. *Understand who you are.* Misalignment between the superintendent's job and their health is an equation for failure, burnout, and moderate to severe health issues. Superintendents must chisel through things that impact their overall performance as a leader and their overall health. You must not try to be someone you are not; it never turns out well. In pursuit of a job, too many superintendents try to become someone they are not, which is the first step for stress, anxiety, and unhealthy work-life balance. Before becoming a superintendent, take time and understand you.

Voices from the Field

Sculpting a Balance Using a Chisel

John Mayfield is a forty-three-year-old male and has been superintendent of a 4,700-student suburban school district in the Midwest for the past six years. There are so many things he enjoys about being a superintendent. John enjoys waking up each morning, arriving at the office, speaking with staff, and then rushing to get into schools and interacting with students, teachers, staff, and principals.

He has an outgoing personality and genuinely enjoys interacting with people. More specifically, he likes to help others. As superintendent he sees himself more as a servant than he does a leader, as he tries to stay in the background and allow others to lead from the front, providing support, encouragement, and resources. Mr. Mayfield prefers to allow others to get credit for the many successes in the district.

Mr. Mayfield's first couple of years were tough, just as they are for many other superintendents. He was prepared to be a superintendent; he did his homework and knew what he was getting into. The problem he experienced from the beginning was that he took on too much. John was involved too much and wanted to be in every meeting, meet everyone, and be as visible as possible, therefore attending every school and community event possible.

He eventually found himself becoming exhausted, working around the clock. He was working long hours, never at home, and rarely made time for himself. He wasn't sleeping, he was eating on the go, and he wasn't exercising as much as he should have been. Prior to becoming a superintendent, Mr. Mayfield took care of himself, but the job, from the beginning, got out of control. Though he was professionally prepared to handle the job, he wasn't personally prepared.

By the end of his first year as superintendent, he had gained almost ten pounds, which really was noticeable. John felt the extra weight, as his knees started giving him problems and he was experiencing chronic stomach issues. Furthermore, he averaged four hours of sleep, as opposed to seven hours before he became superintendent. He felt tired all the time because he was working late and getting up early. He wasn't giving his body enough time at night to rejuvenate. He was trying to lead on a near-empty fuel tank.

The summer after Mr. Mayfield's first year as superintendent, he had to make a personal and professional decision to get his health back. If he expected to have a long tenure as a superintendent, something had to give. He had to come to the realization that he couldn't allow the job to consume all his time if he expected to remain healthy, which is a prerequisite for a long tenure as a superintendent.

Mr. Mayfield had to become realistic about the job—that if he didn't prioritize his schedule each day, identifying what meeting he needed to attend, what decisions he needed to be involved in making, and what event he needed to attend, his health was only going to get worse. He could no longer keep the schedule he had or continue to put his body and mind through this level of stress.

John learned after his first year what his body could and couldn't do. Some superintendents may never discover the importance of a healthy work-life balance. Though it took him a year to discover just how much stress his body and mind could endure, he was fortunate that he only gained weight and experienced stomach issues. He is convinced that if he had not made the decision to use a "chisel" to his schedule, he would have experienced more health conditions.

Like many superintendents, especially first-year superintendents, Mr. Mayfield was afraid to admit he was working too much. He knew in the back of his mind he was working too much and only hurting himself, but he told himself that leaders don't complain. He remembered what his high school basketball coach once said, "When it comes to pain, leaders have to push through it."

He was applying this way of thinking, even though he wasn't pushing through anything. In fact, John was slowing down and experiencing more pain, no matter how hard he tried to overlook what was happening. He was committed to the job, but not so much to his own health. He wrongly believed that he had to choose between the job and his health. He finally discovered that a healthy work-life balance does wonders for his effectiveness as a leader and his overall health.

Now, Mr. Mayfield is a better superintendent for "chiseling" away things of the job. He has learned how to delegate better. More importantly, he has learned how to better navigate the job, while still being visible and accessible. He still attends school and community events, but not every event, as that is when he starts wearing himself down. John realized that he was in a marathon, not a race, and he didn't need to burn himself out on the first stretch if he expected to finish the marathon.

Key Takeaway

There is nothing more important for a superintendent to learn than when to say "no" and "yes," especially when it comes to their schedule.

Superintendents cannot be in every meeting, attend every event, work long hours week after week, and expect to maintain their health. Superintendents must get over the belief that quantity (long hours, more meetings, and events) translates into being more effective.

The best thing you can do, as a superintendent, to be more effective is to make your health and well-being a priority. To do this, you must take a chisel to your job and work to remove or delegate nonessential decisions, events, and meetings, which all tend to impact your health and well-being only negatively, keeping you from being an effective leader. To be an effective leader for the long term, you must let go of some of the weight of the job. Don't be afraid to delegate, prioritize, and focus on yourself!

CHAPTER SIX

Value Your Scars

"Out of suffering have emerged the strongest souls; the most massive characters are seamed with scars."

—Edwin Hubbell Chapin

Due to the nature of the superintendency, it is impossible for a leader not to have scars. If superintendents don't have scars, then chances are they aren't taking risks or doing their job well. Scars are not always visible with leaders; they sometimes are deep, below the surface from previous experiences. On any given day, given the number of decisions a superintendent makes or the number of people they interact with, they are bound to have scars from one of these experiences.

The thing about scars is that they mean that the person survived the ordeal. Scars are reminders that whatever happened yesterday, the superintendent is still leading today. Superintendents often begin to dwell on their scars, questioning if they were worth it, while also developing a sense of anger, which leads to stress, anxiety, and depression. All of these diminish the superintendent's ability to lead effectively.

Depression continues to be on the rise among adults, which also means superintendents are becoming increasingly depressed. As of late, superintendents have had to lead during one of the most difficult and unstable times in education because of a global health pandemic. Likewise, they are leading during a time in which many are experiencing backlash from their communities, decreasing support for elected boards of education, and culture wars.

Undoubtedly, many superintendents will develop scars from this period of education, either small or large.

The key is for superintendents not to dwell on the past or the scars that they developed. It is not healthy. These experiences that lead to scarring are valuable learning experiences for any leader. Though valuable, superintendents can't allow the scars to determine their future, by being fearful of future scars, second-guessing their decisions, or trying to psychoanalyze those who may have led to the scars. The only thing that comes from dwelling on scars is anxiety, stress, timid leadership, and long-term health issues.

In simple terms, a superintendent valuing their scars is one thing, but becoming fixated on the scars and those who may have been involved is not healthy. To be clear, a superintendent, if they are doing their job effectively, really doesn't have time to dwell on the past, yet many do each day. What happened five, ten, or fifteen years ago must be let go if a leader expects to move forward.

There are so many more important things a superintendent can be doing, instead of focusing on the past. There is nothing positive on any level about dwelling in the past. Everyone makes mistakes, develops scars, and has the opportunity to move forward. Those leaders who value their scars and experiences and view them as a learning opportunity and part of life are more effective and healthier.

Stress, nervousness, anxiety, and depression are sub-surface illnesses that are real and often derail many. Leaders must recognize how fast stress can lead to depression. Stress comes with the office. In all honesty, every superintendent experiences some level of stress as they lead school districts, although some more than others. But it is going to happen. So, superintendents must be able to recognize when they are stressed, have a release, and be able to mitigate the amount of stress they experience. It is important that superintendents know their stress points and quickly work to address their stress so it does not lead to short or long-term health issues.

For the sake of their health and well-being, superintendents must change their view toward scars. Scars are just part of the job and life. They are reminders that sometimes a person wins, and sometimes they lose. But more importantly, no matter how painful the scar is or was, it is healed, in the past, and now they must move forward. Superintendents can't lead effectively if they are timid and always trying to avoid pain.

They will find that trying to avoid painful situations or situations that may lead to scarring is just as detrimental to their health. Just lead! Use the past as a learning experience, but move forward—it's healthier. Superintendents must look at their scars every now and then and tell themselves that they are stronger and more effective as a result. Wear it with pride! Scars heal and are not something to continue to dwell on.

Practical Strategies

1. *Reflect regularly.* Reflection, whether in writing or quietly, is transformative. Spending several minutes a day, especially during times of stress, will help lower stress and focus more on the now and less on the past. Reflection is a simple release process that takes little time but is rejuvenating and transformative. Reflection can help you keep from becoming fixated on your scars or the negatives in your life, and help you find a healthy path forward.

2. *Seek counseling for distractions* Though reflecting is an excellent strategy to practice, superintendents may need more expertise in helping them to cope and navigate their health concerns and to stop dwelling on the past. There is nothing wrong with talking to others if it helps the superintendent to find balance. Too often, leaders feel bad or weak by seeking counseling, but let's be honest, the superintendency is not easy. It's extremely complicated. Sometimes the scars are too much to handle alone, and there are excellent experts available to help coach superintendents through the process of addressing their scars and moving forward. If the job or life has become too much, find help and see a counselor who specializes in the field of helping professionals find balance.

3. *Keep pushing forward.* Superintendents must be careful not to fall into the trap of focusing on all the wrongs in their lives or mistakes. This does suggest that they bury themselves in work and ignore the past or their stress. You should always try and focus on the right now positives, making sure that you have a good team that surrounds you at work and that you have a healthy work-life balance. When it comes to a team, make sure that each member also prioritizes their health and well-being too. Scars, stress, or working too much can make you lose focus and begin dwelling on the past, which only leads to more stress, exhaustion, and derailment in the effectiveness of a leader.

Voices from the Field

Scars Hurt, But Are Healthy, If Used Correctly

Dr. Sonya Gupta is a fifty-three-year-old female who has been a superintendent for eight years of a 3,400-student school district in a rural Midwest community. She had a phenomenal career as a substitute teacher, teacher, principal, district administrator, and now as superintendent. She climbed the ladder and had so many experiences that helped her to be effective as superintendent.

Sonya and her family have been blessed in so many ways. Though successful, Sonya has had to take some time to come to the realization that there are so many positives in her life and career. She is one of those that dwelled on the past for many years. She couldn't let go of the past, and it was hindering her ability to navigate the present and future. Like many, though she had thickened skin, deep down, rejection was hard for her.

Her dedication to education has never wavered, but her job performance wasn't the best, especially when she started trying to move up the career ladder. As research shows, being a female makes it a little more difficult to climb the career ladder in education. Most principals and superintendents are males. The superintendency very much remains dominated by males. Like many females who may read this, Sonya endured struggles as she tried to climb the ladder.

Though change is occurring, and more females are breaking through the glass ceiling in education, the process was exceedingly difficult for Dr. Gupta. She lost count of how many times she applied for an administrator position at the school and district level and was beaten out by someone else, a male candidate in most cases. Though she was professionally qualified and had the experience necessary to become a district or school administrator, each time she was overlooked for the job, she began to question her abilities.

Application after application and interview after interview, Sonya's stress level would go up, as well as her internal anger. She would rehash the interview in her head trying to determine what she may have said or how she could have changed her response to a question. The days and weeks after each interview were exceedingly trying on her emotional and mental health. She didn't want to work and became depressed because she felt she was letting her students down. She was not in a good place.

Headaches, nauseousness, severe stomach issues, and anger filled her days and weeks after each interview. Dr. Gupta would allow the fact that she was overlooked for a principalship, a district administrator role, and the superintendency to get to her. That is all she would think about. She questioned her abilities and if she needed to stay in education. Being rejected hurts and leaves a scar. For Sonya, it left multiple. It was consuming her life, personally and professionally. She was depressed and angry at home and at work.

She would eventually become principal and then a district administrator, but it wasn't easy. She put herself through a traumatizing experience each time. For Sonya, climbing the ladder didn't get any easier, even though she thought after becoming a principal, the process for a district administrator and superintendent would be a better experience. It was when she started applying for the superintendency that she knew that she needed help with her health.

Sonya applied for close to ten superintendent vacancies over a three-year period. After the second year, she had made herself so sick that her headaches became chronic, she couldn't eat, and she wanted to sleep all the time. She was so angry with herself and others that she couldn't look past not being hired. It was constantly on her mind, and that is all she wanted to talk about at home with her husband. It was a tough time. She decided to go to a therapist that focused on counseling work-related stress.

Dr. Gupta's therapist was really concerned with how she was processing and viewing each interview process. Her therapist was equally concerned about the impact it was having on Sonya's overall health. Over a period of six months, with weekly sessions, Sonya's therapist helped her to get to a point that allowed her to focus more on all the positives in her life, instead of becoming consumed by all the negatives.

Sonya's therapist helped her realize that she had many more positives than she did negatives in her life. Her therapist said rejection is never easy and never without pain, but that that shouldn't define who Sonya is, personally or professionally. Instead of allowing rejection to control her, her therapist helped her to understand how to use rejection to focus on her positives, instead of the few negatives that may exist in her life.

It wasn't an effortless process. Sonya's therapist helped her to realize that her continual focus on the past and previous interviews were standing in the way of her getting the current job. Her therapist helped her to realize that not getting a job is more about the other candidate, instead of about her. However, Sonya needed to approach each interview with a new sense of excitement and opportunity and not take all the grudges and previous rejections with her into the interview.

Dr. Gupta had to apply for three additional positions before landing her first superintendency. She finally made it, but it wasn't a journey paved in gold. She had to get herself emotionally and mentally ready. She had become so focused on everything wrong in her life that she was overlooking everything that was positive, including her family. For years, her stress was all caused by scars—each rejection she received as she climbed the career ladder. She was allowing herself to be consumed by scars, instead of present opportunities.

Her scars, especially her focus on them, were hindering her personally and professionally. The headaches, nauseousness, and stomach issues that Dr. Gupta experienced were mild considering what would have happened if she did not get help to address her feelings of rejection, anger, and, yes, depression. The hope of Dr. Gupta's story is that it helps someone to work through their scars and look at all the positives that exist in their lives today—they are there!

Key Takeaway

Superintendents are encouraged to wear scars with pride, not as something that they have to hide. They must be open about their past decisions and mistakes. But more importantly, they must be proud of their successes and the good things that they have done. The job of a superintendent is extraordinarily complex and littered with stress mines each day. Undoubtedly, a superintendent is going to make many mistakes over the course of their career. These mistakes cannot continue to be relitigated in the leader's mind. Superintendents must own up to the mistakes, embrace their scars, and move forward.

Superintendents are encouraged to allow their scars to help create a better path forward, which is more rewarding personally and professionally. As a superintendent, you must train yourself to focus on the positives and what is happening today and tomorrow. You must be cognizant of the past as a learning opportunity, but not something that you continue to dwell on—it isn't healthy for you personally or professionally. Constantly focusing on your scars, mistakes from yesterday, or decisions made years ago, will not help you with your career longevity or your health and well-being.

CHAPTER SEVEN

The Importance of Mondays

"Mondays are the start of the workweek which offer new beginnings 52 times a year."

—David Dweck

Mondays are more than just the first day of the workweek. Wait—superintendents work seven days a week! But for this intent and purpose, let's pretend that Monday is the start of the workweek. Mondays are a critical day, not only for professional reasons but also for our well-being. Mondays are typically the first day people attempt to diet, with the mindset, let me enjoy one more weekend eating or drinking what they want, one more weekend to stay glued to the recliner at home, or one more opportunity to stay fixated on the job, not family or my well-being.

Too often, superintendents begin Mondays just like they left off on Friday before, focused solely on the job and paying little attention to their own health and well-being. The workweek for a superintendent blends together; there is no end or start of the workweek. Superintendents push themselves, many to a breaking point, trying to work around the clock, fifty-two weeks per year, and at the end of the year, many look back and seem unfulfilled by their work.

Hence the importance of Mondays. Mondays are new beginnings for superintendents, professionally and personally. They can start another week with a blank slate, with the opportunity to create change for students and employees, as well as for our own health and well-being. Effective superintendents recognize the importance of Mondays as a new beginning. Though many superintendents by Wednesday are looking forward to Friday (everyone does), Mondays are often overlooked as a critical day professionally and personally.

It is hard to get going on Mondays, as everyone feels the drag to start back to work. Superintendents utilize the weekends to recharge or at least recharge for another action-packed, dynamic, and energy-packed week. If a leader doesn't make Monday count, professionally or personally, then the rest of the week never improves. What happens on Monday lasts throughout the week, either positively or negatively.

Ensuring that Mondays are positive is essential not only for a superintendent's effectiveness for the week but also for the effectiveness of the organization. The mood, work ethic, and health of the superintendent are felt throughout the school district. If the superintendent consistently has a "case of Mondays" then everyone else also feels the effects. The goal is to make sure that Mondays are as positive and high-energy as possible. If superintendents can utilize weekends to recharge their minds and bodies, as well as restore their work-life balance, then all prerequisites are met to a positive and action-packed Monday.

Make Mondays count professionally and personally. In terms of health, superintendents who exercise and remain committed to a diet plan on Mondays will more likely finish the work week with the same discipline and dedication to their health. If a superintendent skips their focus on health on Monday, they are less likely to focus on health through Friday. Again, ensuring your Mondays are positive and high-energy is critical to the effectiveness of the leadership position and overall health.

Never underestimate the importance of new beginnings. Mondays offer fresh opportunities to everyone who embraces the opportunity. The key is to make every day leading up to Monday count. Mondays are important; however, there is work involved and a commitment the leader must provide. Monday's can help erase a lot of things, but you can't stop your new journey on Tuesday through Sunday. Mondays are for new beginnings and new journeys, but Tuesday through Sunday is a warmup to prepare you for the opportunities that await Monday.

Practical Strategies

1. *Focus on your schedule.* Superintendents need to make sure that they have time scheduled on Mondays for health and well-being. If they work out, exercise, and remain committed to their diets on Monday, they are more likely to follow through the rest of the week. If you

exercise (walk, run, lift weights, swim, play golf, tennis, etc.) every Monday, your whole week will change. Think about starting your Mondays off focused on health and well-being; you will be refreshed and less likely to have a case of the Mondays!

2. *Use Mondays to try new things.* Mondays are a perfect day for superintendents to try a new workout to spice up their training, experiment with a new diet, or adopt a new work schedule. This will help shock their bodies. Likewise, you are encouraged to start new leadership initiatives or try something new in your job on Mondays. It is recommended that you ensure meetings on Monday are positive, as much as possible. Schedule, when feasible, dreaded meetings on Tuesday through Thursday, keeping Mondays and Fridays focused on setting the mood for the rest of the week. By doing so you can go into the weekend on a positive note.

3. *Prioritize Monday.* Superintendents are encouraged to prioritize their Mondays, making them the healthiest day of the week or the most effective and positive professionally. By making Mondays important, the outlook for the remainder of the week is so much better. Mondays are days to start new workouts, diets, or initiatives. You can use Mondays as a springboard for the rest of the week.

4. *Stay clear of those who always have a case of the Mondays.* Superintendents set the tone for the organization, including the level of positivity and negativity. Negativity is highly contagious, which is why positivity is so important to be modeled by the superintendent. No matter the circumstances or situation, you must remain committed to being positive, energetic, and always eager to start the workweek—and ensuring that others see your positivity and energy and how you prioritize the importance of Mondays.

Voices from the Field

Start the Week Off on a Positive Note

Lydia Rutherford is a fifty-eight-year-old superintendent in her fifth year at a 5,000-student, rural school district in the Southwest. She became superintendent by being in the right place at the right time. She was an assistant superintendent for the district and became interim once the superintendent decided to retire unexpectedly due to a health issue mid-year. She served as interim for approximately six months and was later named the superintendent.

The board of education thought Lydia was doing an excellent job. Furthermore, both Mrs. Rutherford and the board of education enjoyed a positive relationship. She is one of those people who believes that relationships matter, especially the relationship between members of the board of education and the superintendent. Lydia enjoyed being the superintendent, even though she really didn't aspire to become one.

Mrs. Rutherford was perfectly satisfied with being an assistant superintendent. Though satisfied with being an assistant superintendent she felt blessed and grateful for the opportunity to serve her community, as she was from the community and worked in the district her entire career. Over her career as an educator, she focused on making Mondays count. In Lydia's classroom when she was a high school teacher, she had a weekly calendar posted every week with Monday circled and "make it count" written across the top with the arrow pointing to Mondays.

Mondays were important to Lydia as a leader. She would always make sure that she was in school first thing on Mondays, ensuring that schools started off the week on a positive note. Mrs. Rutherford told principals to do the same when it comes to Mondays—make it count. She communicated to them that she expected them in classrooms, not sitting behind the desk on Mondays. She would try to model the expectation that Mondays are important to the rest of the week.

On a personal side note, Lydia would work out four to five times per week at home, but she would never miss Monday. She would wake up early and hit the treadmill, weights, or attend a HIIT class at school, offered by one of the physical education teachers in the community. She found that if she exercised on Mondays, she was more likely to work out at least four to five times per week. Mondays were her launchpad personally and professionally. Lydia felt weird the rest of the week if she missed her Monday workout. She would prioritize her calendars to make Mondays count.

Something Mrs. Rutherford also learned over her career is that if Mondays are positive, the rest of the week is also positive. Sure, there would be things that would pop up from time to time that would try to derail her and her schedule, but she was very guarded about Mondays. She would move anything that she felt would start the rest of the week off on the wrong foot to midweek. Lydia preferred not to get trapped in her office any day of the week but especially not on Mondays. Mondays were important to her own well-being, personally and professionally.

Lydia would always look forward to Monday mornings, as she had her entire career, to make Mondays the most important day of the week. She enjoyed Fridays, Saturdays, and Sundays, but Monday was the day that determined the success of the other six days of the week. If her Mondays were stressful, negative, or low energy, the other six days were also stressful, negative, and low energy. She worked to make sure that Mondays are as positive as they can be. It was overwhelming, at least to her, to think about seven days, therefore, she would focus on one—Mondays, which impacts all the other days.

Key Takeaway

There is one day that matters the most, and that day is Monday. So many people are stressed about Mondays because they have not prioritized the day. Mondays are going to determine how positive, enjoyable, and healthy the rest of the week is for a superintendent. As mentioned throughout this book, the superintendency is stressful. Therefore, anything that can be done to lower the stress should be done. If Mondays are stressful, then the rest of the week is also more than likely going to be stressful.

Superintendents must always start their Mondays focused on their own health and well-being. The job can't always consume everything in their lives. Monday is the day that they must make sure that to do something that focuses on their health and well-being, like physical movement—lifting weights, walking, running, aerobics, or swimming. You must get your body and mind acclimated for the workweek. Focus on being positive and improving your health and well-being, and the results will be transformative. Though a lot of people focus on rushing to Friday, Saturday, and Sunday, understandably so, making Monday important and positive will make those other three days even more exciting.

CHAPTER EIGHT

The Rejuvenating Walkabout

"Walking is man's best medicine."

—Hippocrates

One of the best stress-relief and well-being strategies is to walk daily. Walking reduces stress, strengthens the immune system, and improves a person's overall view of themselves. As few as twenty minutes of walking each day is transformative in a big way, no matter if the superintendent is active, athletic, or doesn't exercise at all. Superintendents need to stop and think about lowering their stress levels and improving their effectiveness as leaders by just allocating minutes each day to walk.

Understandably, many superintendents will ask themselves how they can walk each day based on their schedule. However, squeezing in a few minutes each day is easier than one may think. Too many superintendents are trying to lead behind their desks by utilizing telephones, virtual chats, and memos. Superintendents cannot lead effectively from behind a desk or through memos.

Employees, students, and the community need superintendents to be seen in their districts. Repeatedly, we hear that the community wants a superintendent who is on the frontline. They are not paying for someone to sit behind a desk and dictate orders. In comes the power of walking. In districts where superintendents are accessible and visible, they experience higher student and teacher engagement, which leads to higher student achievement and improved teacher effectiveness.

Though superintendents may not feel comfortable with scheduling their daily walk on their calendars for others to see, it's imperative to their own health and well-being to do so. But instead of marking down "daily walk," why not write down "walkthroughs," which is an essential part of the job. No matter the school district size, superintendents should visit at least one school each day and five classrooms. Remember, blocking off twenty to thirty minutes is minimal but can be transformative. Superintendents are killing two birds with one stone by visiting schools; being accessible to employees, students, and the community; and also focusing on their well-being.

There is a debate on how long a walkthrough should be performed. It all depends on the focus of the superintendent's walkthrough. Is the walk-through focused on teaching and learning, operations, and culture? A good rule of thumb is to allocate at least fifteen to twenty minutes per classroom. Though most of the walkthroughs are observation and listening, with each step superintendents add to their total walking minutes while also carrying out a key function of the superintendency—being accessible and visible.

To be clear, walking each day is imperative for superintendents' health. With each step, superintendents are doing so many positive things for their overall health and well-being. Yes, superintendents are always focused on organizational performance, like other leaders, but walkabouts are also a necessity for the superintendent's health. No matter the superintendent's age, they need to be walking daily, not being sedentary for extended periods of time throughout the day, which leads to poor blood circulation, obesity, increased stress, and other serious health conditions.

There is absolutely nothing wrong with performing walkabouts as a super-intendent. More importantly, there is nothing wrong with a superintendent making their own health and well-being a priority. Superintendents will find themselves more productive, present, and positive by performing walkabouts each day. Too many superintendents will try to make an excuse that they can't find time to focus on their own health. Well, walkabouts help solve this problem and do not interfere with their job. Furthermore, walking is simple, free, and highly transformative, both personally and professionally.

In today's schools, it is impossible for a superintendent to be effective by staying fixed behind a desk. Superintendents must keep their fingers on the pulse of the district. There is no better way to feel and observe the culture of the district than by walking through the school district, observing and listening, with extraordinarily little talking. Keep in mind, the purpose of the walkthrough is to connect with employees, students, and the community, while the superintendent also makes a connection to their own well-being.

Practical Strategies

1. *Schedule walkabouts.* Superintendents should choose a time each day, for instance, mid-morning around 10:00 a.m. and right after lunch around 1:00 p.m. for walkabouts. Around 10:00 a.m. and the hour right after lunch is typically when educators begin to feel the effects of their energy dropping. Their energy begins to fade, they feel tired, and they need a boost of energy to make it the rest of the day. Plus, especially after lunch, walking helps to improve digestion.

2. *Prioritize walking.* Throughout the day, superintendents should be looking to schedule at least fifteen to thirty minutes of walking each day. This can include visiting classrooms, speaking and listening to staff, and checking facilities and grounds. The most important thing is that you are moving and not staying sedentary for the entire workday. You must force yourself to walk and schedule opportunities to walk and move throughout your day. This should be in addition to your daily exercise routine.

3. *Track your steps.* Superintendents' walking goals should be 10,000-plus steps each day. Though there is no research behind the 10,000 steps per day goal, tracking their steps will tell superintendents how much they move or sit during the day. You should always move more than you sit during the day. A good rule of thumb is for every forty-five minutes a superintendent is sitting behind their desk or around a table meeting, they should walk at least fifteen minutes. For instance, if you have been in a meeting for 45 minutes, make sure that you have fifteen minutes immediately afterward to walk around the office or outside to help with blood circulation.

4. *Stand and work.* Increasingly superintendents are opting for standing desks instead of sitting behind a desk. Standing, instead of sitting, helps blood circulation, concentration, and helps to give you more energy. If you can't seem to find time to perform walkthroughs or walk throughout the day, think about purchasing a standing desk. The results will be transformative.

Voices from the Field

Walking for Health and the Ability to Lead

Dr. Sally Ford is a fifty-six-year-old superintendent of an urban school district in the Northwest in her seventh year. There are so many things about the superintendency that are designed to keep superintendents behind their desks for hours at a time if they are not careful. All superintendents know or have known superintendents who try to lead their districts from behind their desks, using email, phone calls, text, or memos.

Though leading an organization from behind the desk may have worked decades ago, it is not an effective leadership strategy for superintendents to follow today. The problems of sitting behind a desk the entire workday go far beyond the leadership position. It is unhealthy for anyone to sit the entire day. Sally remembers from personal experience that when her father experienced his first stroke, his doctor kept telling him after each doctor visit that for every forty-five minutes that he sat at home reading the newspaper or watching his favorite television show, he should get up and walk outside for at least fifteen minutes to help improve his blood circulation. Sadly, Sally's father didn't listen and suffered numerous strokes before finally passing away from a massive one.

The doctor's message of walking really resonated with Dr. Ford, especially since she discovered that strokes ran in her family. Prior to learning about the importance of walking, she too was sitting too much throughout the day and not moving enough. Like many superintendents, she would get trapped behind her desk signing documents, responding to emails, drafting correspondence, or sitting in meetings. Sally discovered it was quite easy to get trapped behind her desk.

After her father passed away, Sally started really paying attention to how long she stayed seated behind her desk or at a conference table. She worked closely with her administrative assistant to organize her schedule. One strategy she started using to get her moving more throughout the day was to schedule many classroom walkthroughs or school visits each day and schedule them throughout the day. By visiting classrooms and schools, yes, she was monitoring what is occurring in the district, but she was also addressing her own health.

As one can imagine, her overall mood changed after her walkthroughs. After a stressful meeting, Dr. Ford would go for a walk—visiting the bus garage, visiting a classroom, checking the district's grounds, or just walking around the parking lot—focusing on breathing and clearing her mind. With each step, she was able to get her mental and physical health in balance. This will be hard for many superintendents, as they are overwhelmed and being pulled in so many directions each day. Many become stressed just trying to understand how to prioritize their health.

What Sally learned is that she had to make her health part of the job. She felt that making her health a priority only helped her to become a better leader. Her focus on her health does not compromise her ability to lead and she has not missed a meeting or jeopardized anything operationally in the district by going for a walk. After she started walking, the staff noticed how she was more present in meetings and one-on-one conversations. One staff member told her, after a couple of months of walking, to keep doing whatever she was doing because she was more positive, happier, and more accessible to staff.

Dr. Ford's commitment to walking required a walking routine that did not occur overnight. It took her several months to figure out the best way to walk throughout the day. After several years, she is now walking at least one hour a day, but on a good day, she's rarely behind her desk. One additional trick she used was to install a standing desk in her office where she stands as she responds to emails, drafts memos, joins virtual meetings, or answers phone calls.

The standing desk was a notable change for her and for the district office, as other staff, once they saw her new desk, wanted one as well. People who she knew sat 100 percent of the day were suddenly standing for most of the day. So, Sally's focus on her health has trickled down to others. That's a win-win for her and the district. It is important for superintendents not to allow the job to control their health. Superintendents cannot fall victim to the idea that they don't have time to go for a walk, because that is simply not true.

Like many superintendents, Dr. Ford struggled at first, but she pushed forward and stopped worrying about what people may think if they saw her walking too much or found her out of her office. She finally had to come to grips with the fact that if she didn't move consistently every day, her health was going to be impacted. She resolved that if her health was impaired, then she couldn't lead effectively.

It took some time for Dr. Ford to understand how important her health was to her ability to lead. Though her change in thinking didn't happen overnight, she now wouldn't change her schedule or how she leads. She strongly recommends that other superintendents start small at first but make sure that they move each day . . . every day. But she also encourages her staff to move throughout the day. As a result, the entire culture at the district office has changed, and more importantly, the culture has become healthier.

Key Takeaway

Leading effectively requires a leader to be healthy. Sitting behind a desk all day is no longer going to allow the leader to effectively lead. More importantly, sitting behind a desk for most of the day is going to have a significant, negative impact on the superintendent's health. Changing the mindset of many superintendents today, that they can lead from behind the desk and never leave their office, will be hard. But this change must occur.

Like with anything, start small and with a plan. Walking doesn't take a lot to have a transformative effect on a person's health. The superintendent's job description has many avenues that can lead to someone moving throughout the workday. Superintendents have many opportunities throughout the day to walk if they evaluate their job and what is expected of them. Most boards of education and communities want a superintendent who is visible and accessible in the district; visiting classrooms, walking the school grounds, or walking to meetings in the community are good for their job and, more importantly, for their health.

CHAPTER NINE
The Healing and Rejuvenating Power of Faith

"Faith and prayer are the vitamins of the soul; man cannot live in health without them."

—Mahalia Jackson

Faith is rarely discussed in terms of well-being and even more seldom with school leadership. Though many school superintendents have faith and indicate that they pray, neither is thought of to improve well-being. There must be a certain level of faith among school superintendents. The job continues to become more complex, which undoubtedly causes more stress. Superintendents must have faith in themselves and something greater if they expect to be successful.

Faith and prayer can help to lower stress. Doctors prescribe prayer a lot to medical patients in hospitals, even the most severely ill, so there must be something to it if leading physicians are utilizing it. Some of the job responsibilities are simply too much for one person to handle. The superintendency is a lonely position, especially in smaller school districts and communities.

So as the stresses of the job continue to increase, superintendents often don't have others to turn to discuss, reflect, and lower stress. When speaking with superintendents, many, especially those superintendents who are in incredibly stressful positions, indicate that they pray regularly and feel better about themselves for doing so. For just a few minutes, superintendents are able to step away from hectic and stressful moments of the job, which happens regularly.

There is something about faith and prayer for leaders. Though there is next to no research that connects prayer, faith, and well-being to the superintendency, there are superintendents that wear their faith—based on a quick search on social media. Prayer helps superintendents to reach a certain level of peace about and confidence in their decision or the outcomes. This level of peace leads to less stress, which helps to improve the overall health of superintendents. With prayer, leaders stop trying to please everyone, are less likely to make erratic decisions, and become more connected with their own leadership style and spirituality.

Faith allows superintendents to realize that life is full of struggle, and they must have a certain level of faith to navigate the many curveballs that are thrown at them daily. Faith allows superintendents to believe in something bigger than the job, in the abilities of others, and that at the end of the day everything finds a balance, no matter how good or bad the day is.

When superintendents realize that they are not alone, that they are bigger and greater forces in charge, a sense of relief falls on superintendents. Superintendents who seldom pray, have lost faith, or indicate no faith at all, are more likely to have a shorter tenure as a district leader. The pressures and stresses of the job are just too much for superintendents to handle and carry alone. Throughout the day the number of decisions made, obstacles faced, or stressors experienced are overwhelming to the most seasoned superintendent. So much so that each day the health and well-being of superintendents take direct hits that if not addressed can and often do lead to serious health issues, if not recognized or left untreated.

Prayer takes very little time during the day compared to other things personally and professionally. Superintendents who make this a constant calendar event seem to be more energized, less stressed, and healthier. Furthermore, they are more present in the job and can lead more effectively. Prayer is an easy, quick, and free stress reliever that can lead to better health and well-being. Prayer is transformative for the body, mind, soul, and profession. Superintendents are faced with so many things each day, and prayer is a relief strategy that not only relieves stress but also instills a sense of hope and faith, even during the darkest and most stressful days of the job.

Practical Strategies

1. *Start and end the day with prayer or reflection.* If a superintendent is not a "praying" type, that's no problem. They should reflect on their day. This is an opportunity to reflect on the positives and negatives of the day and plan the next day. It's amazing how prayer and reflection are

transformative for the mind and soul. You can spend five to ten minutes separated from the job and focused only on yourself.

2. *Take occasional breaks during stressful moments.* Ideally, superintendents have carved out time during the workday to spend time alone. Though some days prayer and reflection may seem impossible, leaders need this time. There is nothing wrong with superintendents having a standing block of time in their daily calendar for prayer and reflection. You may call it something different on their calendars, but this is your time to disconnect from the job for a few minutes to reconnect with yourself.

3. *Practice prayer daily.* Prayer, a way to relieve stress and improve well-being, only works when it is regular and consistent, just like exercise. Daily time spent praying and reflecting has rejuvenating qualities for the mind, body, and soul—all three of which directly impact the health and well-being of a superintendent. You may struggle with this, but finding five to ten minutes each day, even before leaving for work, to pray, meditate, and reflect, will help.

4. *Be comfortable with faith, prayer, and reflection.* Superintendents don't need to hide the fact that they have faith, pray, meditate, or reflect. Hiding who they are is counterproductive to improving their well-being. This isn't about praying in public; this is about recognizing the transformative power of faith and prayer. Spending time reflecting and praying are highly personal, and in order to be transformative must be tailored to the comfort level of the superintendent. Some may choose to be more public than others, and that's okay, but you must choose what works for you.

Voices from the Field

Overlooking What Matters the Most: Faith and Hope

Rachel Schumer is a sixty-year-old superintendent, serving the past twelve years in a suburban school district in the Midwest. Many superintendents work to the point they lose faith, not only in themselves but also in others and in God. If they haven't, they are blessed. Rachel is one of the superintendents who lost faith and now feels embarrassed, ashamed, and afraid it will happen again.

Several years ago, she became so immersed in her job that she couldn't tell whether she was at home or at the office. It seemed as if Rachel was bringing work home, steadily increasing the amount of work each week. It wasn't that she didn't do work at the office, she was. She couldn't get everything accomplished, so she felt it necessary to take her work home with her each night.

After about six months of doing this, her schedule really changed. You see, prior to becoming a superintendent, Mrs. Schumer considered herself a church-going person who believed in faith and had hope. Every Sunday morning, she was there and regularly attended Bible study on Wednesday night. But that changed. It started with Mrs. Schumer missing church every now and then, and eventually grew to her never attending church.

She couldn't find time to breathe much less spend two hours at church on Sunday mornings. She was so swamped at work that she gave up something that really meant a lot to her. After stopping going to church and praying, she lost a sense of direction and let her health go. All Rachel was doing was working and eating, with extraordinarily little sleep. Though this may seem overly dramatic, she wished it didn't happen.

Rachel gained weight, developed dark bags under her eyes, and started to experience severe headaches. She would wake up in the morning not feeling rested. Her days and weeks seemed to be running together. She felt she didn't have time to breathe, eat lunch, or disconnect from the job. Her work was consuming every waking minute. Throughout the day her eyes would fill with tears of exhaustion.

She kept asking herself how she let her life get so out of balance. She considered herself a strong female leader, but honestly, she was ineffective a couple of years ago. She learned the hard way that the number of hours at work does not equate to effective leadership, but rather, extremely poor health. Rachel eventually got her life back to normal. It took her several months of medical appointments to finally realize that if something didn't change, her hope of a brighter day would quickly fade from the horizon.

Rachel finally returned to Sunday morning services and Bible study on Wednesday evenings, rejuvenated by faith, and decided to cut back on work. It wasn't easy. Now several years have passed, and she is still at peace with her life. She can finally breathe and enjoy doing things she likes to do. Members of the board of education and her colleagues tell her that she is a better leader now and seems happier.

Key Takeaway

Something so simple, easy, and free is exceedingly difficult to do. It's always the simple things in life that we often miss. Superintendents must prioritize their schedules each day based on the on-the-ground needs of the day. Superintendents are pulled in so many different directions each day, there is no surprise that many eventually indicate that they are stressed to the limit, exhausted, or burned out, especially because of the past several years navigating the complexities of school during a global health pandemic.

Though the job is so stressful, superintendents must have a consistent, simple, and accessible relief. Prayer, reflection, and faith are free, accessible from any location, and simple. The only thing that is required of the superintendent is time. Though time is a precious commodity for any superintendent, prayer only requires a few minutes each day to be transformative. You don't have to go to a gym, outside, or to a designated spot to pray. It can be done anywhere that you can be alone—the office, outdoors, or in a vehicle.

If you reflect on the day, think how often you are in the office, outside, or driving around in your vehicle. All are perfect opportunities to stop for five to ten minutes to pray, reflect, and breathe. If it is important to you, the leader, then you will prioritize your schedule no matter what it is—meeting with board members, community or business leaders, teachers, or attending a budget meeting. All of these are important, but nothing is more important than prioritizing time for your health and well-being, so allocating a few minutes during the workday for you to pray, meditate, and reflect doesn't seem so far-fetched.

CHAPTER TEN

Disconnect to Connect More . . . With Yourself

"In a world of algorithms, hashtags and followers, know the true importance of human connection."

—Simi Froman

Tens, if not hundreds of emails and text messages clog a superintendent's inbox or cellphone. On many days, superintendents find themselves looking at a screen on their computer or laptop or their cellphones. The goal of accessibility has moved the superintendency more dependent on technology, instead of face-to-face interactions and communications. As superintendents become more mobile, rarely in their office, the need for around-the-clock connectivity will grow, as the importance of media devices will only increase in need.

Though superintendents remain connected to the job, more specifically to their communication toolbox that consists of their cellphones and laptop, they actually become more disconnected with other important things such as their health, family, friends, and coworkers. We have all seen people walking around at the local supermarket, in a team meeting, in the office, or at home, glued to their cellphones. It seems as if there is no downtime for anyone these days. But as we prioritize our connectivity, we continue to create lasting damage to our overall health and well-being.

It is not healthy to look at a computer screen or cell phone screen every five minutes. Mentally, emotionally, and physically, the more we look at electronic screens the more we become shackled to stress. Sure, not all texts or emails bring unwelcome news or require another decision that must be made, but when we fail to give our eyes and brain a rest, stress develops. Stress will start small, but it becomes a snowball out of control quickly.

Superintendents often go to bed looking at their cell phones updating, or reading social media, or checking and responding to texts and emails. The minute they wake up in the morning, most superintendents indicate they check their phones first thing, and when they go to bed at night, they check their phones one last time. This is all occurring while sleep patterns for leaders continue to decrease. Forget seven or eight hours of sleep each night; it is more like four to five hours per night due to their schedule. Superintendents do not have time to recharge each night, to give their eyes and minds a break, as they stay connected to their mobile devices.

As meetings have steadily required the usage of virtual technologies and presentations, leaders and employees remain attached to their desktops or laptops. Newsflash, a virtual meeting or an in-person meeting where everyone is looking at their laptop or desktop screens does not equate to engagement or connection. From a professional standpoint, when an organization values electronic or paper-based communication over face-to-face communications, their culture begins to take a hit. Leaders and employees need those face-to-face interactions to remain connected to the organization and the team. It never hurts for a leader to favor and model face-to-face communication and interactions.

On a personal level, superintendents need to put their phones away and power down their laptops not only for the job but also for their own health and family. When a superintendent is healthy and has a healthy home life, their overall effectiveness improves. Likewise, when a superintendent is unhealthy or has an unhealthy or stressful home life, their overall effectiveness declines. Though many believe that there is no way to balance home and work, it can be done, and the first step is to disconnect from the job more often and reconnect with oneself and their families and friends. Though the demands and pressures that superintendents face are great and seem endless, reconnecting with something positive, healthy, and essential such as family and friends, is transformative to their overall health and their effectiveness as a leader.

Practical Strategies

1. *Disconnect from mobile email.* Superintendents must force themselves to check email a few times throughout the workday. Superintendents must lead and train themselves and their staff to prioritize their communication, preferring face-to-face communication over electronic

communication. If there is something important, then people need to find each other, instead of cluttering inboxes with irrelevant emails that could have been handled face-to-face. But superintendents who stay glued to their email either on their cell phone or their laptop is not an option if they expect to maintain any sanity and well-being.

2. *Set parameters with technology.* Superintendents, in meetings, during meals, and during time with friends and family, should silence their cell phones or leave them on a table, in a bag, or in their vehicle. This will allow them to be more present in meetings, at home, and out with friends. Again, if there is something important, people will find them; there is no need to continue waiting for a text ping, a call vibration or ring, or an email notification. Technology shouldn't control your life or your career, but it can if not kept in check.

3. *Disconnect at a certain time during the day.* Superintendents should not check their email or text messages after a certain point after they get home. You are encouraged to stay away from texting or responding to texts after a designated time. You shouldn't rush to check your email, texts, or social media in the mornings either. You must give your brain and eyes a break from technology as much as you can. Superintendents have become programmed to try to respond as quickly as possible to a text, email, or message, but all this does is consume valuable time that takes away from your health, well-being, leading, family, and friends.

4. *Set meeting norms in which no technology is allowed.* Superintendents must encourage and prioritize face-to-face communications. Develop the expectation for meeting that there is nothing more important to your team than the meeting and personal interactions. As the superintendent, you model the way on this one. Model leaving your phone on your desk or putting it away during meetings and get back to face-to-face communications. Be more present in meetings, not consumed by waiting for the next text, call, or email.

Voices from the Field

Connected but Disconnected from Opportunities

Dr. Patty Ludlow is a forty-three-year-old female and has been superintendent of a medium-sized school district on the East Coast for nine years. She can't believe she is working on her sixth year as superintendent. She never imagined becoming an administrator, much less a superintendent. All she wanted to do growing up was to become an elementary teacher, and, yes, she was excited about having her summers off.

Like many educators, having summers off remains a dream for Patty, as she attends professional development and conferences for betterment. But one day she hopes to enjoy the summer. When she became superintendent, she was surprised by how often her cell phone rang, she received a text notification, or an email popped in her inbox. As a teacher and principal, she had not experienced this level of connectivity. It seemed now as superintendent she was receiving some notification on her cellphone at least every five minutes.

Over the past two years, Patty has really focused on disconnecting from phones, emails, and social media as much as possible. She remembers during her first three years as superintendent how she always had her cellphone in her hand. She had been convinced that she had to remain connected to the job twenty-four hours a day, 365 days a year. No matter what time of day it was, her phone was close by.

On vacation, before the development of waterproof cell phones and waterproof cases, she would carry her Blackberry around in a ziplock bag to the pool or the beach. She freely admits that she would consider herself addicted to her cell phone. Without noticing, at home watching television, helping her kids with homework, or in meetings at the office, she constantly looks down at her phone.

It is so easy to become addicted to connectivity. Dr. Ludlow was afraid not to have her cellphone with her, as she may miss a call from a board member, an email from a teacher, or a social media post. What if there was an emergency at one of the schools? There were a lot of what ifs that convinced her that she needed her cell phone all the time. It got so bad that she ended up with two phones, just in case the battery died on one, she had an emergency phone ready to use.

The breaking point was at dinner one evening with her husband and two kids. They were at a restaurant on a Friday evening, one of those rare Friday evenings in the school year when there wasn't an athletic event. The entire evening, she was glued to her phone, as earlier that day she had been dealing with a major personnel matter. She was answering emails and texts and speaking with the board attorney. She can't remember what she ordered at the restaurant or what her husband or kids ordered.

Later that night Patty's husband told her she was unresponsive to him and the kids the entire night. She would respond with short answers, but nothing was ever meaningful. They had conversations that she was not aware of because she had her head down the entire night looking at her phone or talking on the phone. She had to use her second cell phone because her battery died on her primary phone. She was one of those who usually noticed other people in restaurants who were using their phones, but that night she was one of them.

Dr. Ludlow felt so bad that her family was living their lives without her because she was so engrossed in the work that she couldn't spare five minutes to ask her kids how their day at school was at the restaurant. She knew something had to change, and her husband told her something had to change. He was incredibly supportive but was tired of looking at her with her head down and eyes glued to her cellphone.

Patty's husband told her it is not healthy to look at a screen that long. During her first year, she developed regular headaches that up to the point of becoming a superintendent she seldom experienced. Her husband also said she was also doing permanent damage to her neck, because she was always looking down at her cellphone. But he was adamant that their children rarely participated in family time like they did before she became a superintendent.

The past two years have really been rejuvenating for Dr. Ludlow, her health, and her relationship with her family. Now, she has only one cell phone, which is a major accomplishment. She limits her screen time and never brings her cell phone to the dining table. She made a conscious decision that this was her time with her family. She grew tired of making her family the second priority.

At work, she rarely checks her email on her phone, only checking when she occasionally sits down behind her desk, as she enjoys being in classrooms. Furthermore, Patty monitors her screen time through her cell phone's tracking feature, and over the past two years it has dropped considerably. She has turned her cell phone into somewhat of an "only in the event of an emergency" use device.

What Dr. Ludlow has discovered about limiting her cellphone use and not trying to respond in real time to every email or text message is that she is more present at home and at work. People say that she is more attentive to their questions and conversations. Her kids can talk to her about their day, and she can carry on a meaningful conversation with her husband, making eye contact. Patty's husband told her that he missed seeing her eyes. The job of a superintendent is hard, but it should never make someone choose between the job and their family. Superintendents can disconnect and connect more with the things that really matter to them, including their families and themselves.

Key Takeaway

Society has made everyone, not just superintendents, believe that constant connectivity is essential or required. Society is spending less and less time interacting and talking face to face, opting, preferring, or settling for electronic communication or virtual interactions. This is leading to increased stress and a sense of disconnection from reality, which is not good for a superintendent's health and well-being.

Though the pressures of remaining connected to our cellphones and emails only grow in intensity, there are some superintendents who are choosing to disconnect to be better leaders, husbands, wives, and parents. Additionally, they are choosing to maintain a healthy well-being and balance between work and life. So, it can be done, but it may be hard at first. The key is to prioritize what is important, delegate, and establish boundaries and expectations regarding the superintendency.

Prioritize face-to-face communication over virtual or electronic communication as much as possible. Make sure everyone understands your boundaries regarding when to email or text, because after a certain time at night or during a certain point of the day you should not be responding to an email or text. Never apologize for not having your cellphone during family time or your time. Don't be afraid to put your cellphone in a different room while having dinner with your family or when you are exercising, reflecting, praying, or reading. As you disconnect, notice how more present you are and how you can connect more with those who matter most.

CHAPTER ELEVEN

Don't Believe You Must
Have All the Answers

"There is nothing wrong with making mistakes and not having all the answers, so long as we are willing to admit this and strive for personal betterment. Those who think they know it all have no way of finding out that they don't."

—Leo Buscaglia

Superintendents are expected to make decisions, to lead, to comfort, and to be visionary. As problems arise, they are looked to for answers, solutions, and a path to greener fields. The job places a large burden on the shoulders of superintendents, considering most superintendents are the only district-wide leader in their communities, especially in rural and geographically distant areas. They may be the only centralized leader that those communities have.

Just as physicians, ministers, and elected leaders are looked to for answers, superintendents also are looked to have the answers to questions and solutions to problems. On any given day, a superintendent may have to make tens or hundreds of decisions depending on the day and the size of the district. No matter the size of the district, however, the burden is there for superintendents of small, medium, or large districts.

Superintendents begin to worry about not having the right answer to questions and about having solutions to all the issues that they confront. This pressure to have all the answers eventually begins to chip away at the leader's overall well-being. Headaches, fatigue, loss of sleep, and regular illness begin to be regular occurrences. Eventually, as these things happen more often, the overall effectiveness of the superintendents begins to fade.

Though superintendents are chief executive officers of a complex organization, they cannot possibly have all the answers to the problems that arise or the questions that are asked. Boards of education do not hire superintendents with the idea that they can solve all the problems and have answers to all the questions. This belief that superintendents must have all the answers is typically self-generated. Superintendents try not to panic and pretend to know what to do, all in the name of being a school leader. But these pressures can bemextremely problematic and damaging to one's health.

High-performing or effective superintendents not only do not have all the answers, but they are quick to tell everyone they do not. They are comfortable in their own leadership and realize that not having all the answers does not weaken their abilities to lead but strengthens their position. Others respect them for not pretending. Overall, not worrying about having all the answers helps maintain healthy well-being and not experience the burnout that those superintendents who claim to have all the answers often do.

A superintendent can only extend their tenure as a superintendent if they are able to maintain their health and well-being. Too many superintendents last only a few years because of their health, while others leave due to their leadership abilities and relationships with the board. Pretending to possess all the answers is not healthy for any leader—aspiring, novice, or veteran. It is acceptable and recommended for superintendents to let everyone know that though they may not know everything, they are not afraid to ask others who may have the answers. By doing so, the superintendent's ability to lead is strengthened as their well-being remains healthy.

Practical Strategies

1. *Let everyone know, from the beginning, that you do not have all the answers.* Being honest with everyone does not compromise the superintendent's leadership but strengthens it. You, as the leader, are encouraged to let people know that although you do not have all the answers, you do have the work ethic and humility to ask others for help. Be careful not to place yourself in a situation that makes people believe you have all the answers. This will only lead to you experiencing regular failure and constant stress.

2. *Be willing and comfortable in your own leadership to seek help from others.* Though superintendents may not have all the answers, others will respect the fact they are willing to ask others for help. Furthermore, this will also pay huge dividends toward your health. Though the superintendency brings with it a certain level of stress, the leader

believing they must have all the answers only compounds the stress, which can be damaging to them personally and professionally. Asking for help shows strength and confidence and helps to lower the unnecessary pressures and stresses on your health and well-being.

3. *Develop a group of close advisors, mentors, or friends that you can rely on when situations arise.* This close group of advisors, mentors, and friends will help superintendents both personally and professionally. The superintendent, knowing that this group of mentors, advisors, and friends has their back, experiences less pressure. If you believe that you must always have the answers or solutions, you are unnecessarily taxing your health and well-being. Empower and rely on others for help.

Voices from the Field

Right Answer, Wrong Strategy

Theresa Jackson is a sixty-year-old, seventh-year superintendent of a suburban school district located in the lower Midwest. She remembers her first day on the job, full of energy, excitement, and limitless possibilities. All superintendents start with these three things, but there is one that isn't often discussed. Yes, the pressure to have all the answers to every question asked.

Superintendents are the chief executive officers of large organizations. Why wouldn't they have all the answers? Theresa really struggled with trying to make sure she had all the answers. Each morning she walked into the office, she was ready to help and answer questions. She braced herself each day to be ready for anything and willing to roll up her sleeves to help wherever she was needed.

Mrs. Jackson considers herself self-confident and has always had high self-esteem. She often tells colleagues and aspiring superintendents her first year really took a toll on her self-confidence and her health. She felt that she needed to project confidence no matter the situation, but what she came to realize was that that is extremely difficult, driving her to the point of exhaustion. She would get to the office around 7:00 a.m. and not leave until 6:00 p.m. or 7:00 p.m., on a good day. After 5:00 p.m., she still had four hours of work left due to after-school events and meetings.

Trying to project confidence wears heavily on the body and mind. When a leader is already working to the point of exhaustion, they are doubling the stress on their body, mind, and soul. Theresa never felt refueled in the morning, as she would only get between three and four hours of sleep each night. She knew she wasn't getting enough rest but felt like she had no other choice.

Eventually, Theresa's exhaustion started to seep through. Her co-workers and husband knew something was wrong with her. She made herself sick. Some days she couldn't go to work. She had reached a point of exhaustion that was debilitating. Depression, headaches, nauseousness, and fatigue were all signs that Mrs. Jackson had reached her limit. Though she was giving the job everything she had, she was not taking into consideration her health.

Most new superintendents, no matter how confident they may be, will begin to second guess a decision, answer a question that they may not fully understand, make several mistakes, and always expect to be "okay." This doesn't include constant negative social media posts, newspaper headlines, or countless emails. All of these will wear anyone down. As most superintendents remember, first-year superintendents are drinking water from a fire hydrant.

Luckily, Theresa had a friend and mentor who was a successful former superintendent. She eventually started calling him daily to figure out how to cope with her anxiety about having to have all the answers. Her mentor provided her with some excellent advice and guidance. He first started by recognizing that Theresa's self-confidence and the pressures of trying to have all the answers are misaligned.

Her mentor helped her to understand that she could still be self-confident and portray confidence by saying she didn't have all the answers. Her mentor said that he realized there is an added pressure of being a female superintendent and trying to have all the answers so that others would respect her and the position. However, pretending to have all the answers or stressing about having all the right answers is not a strategy for longevity in the position.

Ms. Jackson began speaking with her mentor every day for the first month. She recollects that she may have called him two or three times a day. Without her mentor, Theresa tells people she would have quit after the first year. Her peace of mind started to gradually return, and her anxiety about going to work slowly went away. She had to train her brain that saying, "I don't have all the answers," did not mean she was an ineffective leader or wasn't confident.

As Mrs. Jackson reflects, she was placing too much pressure on herself to have all the right answers. Now, she always tells people that she doesn't have all the right answers, but she does know people who may. She has empowered others in the office to step up to the plate and help to answer the questions. Instead of going home at night worrying about tomorrow and having knots in her stomach due to anxiety, she goes home more relaxed and looking forward to tomorrow.

It took health issues for Mrs. Jackson to make her realize that her trying to have all the answers only weakens her as a leader. Relying on others to help solve problems and answer questions made her a better, healthier, and more collaborative leader. Superintendents are incredible individuals who want to lead. This does not mean that they must jeopardize their own health just to appear to have all the right answers and to look confident. It is not a strategy that results in a long tenure as a superintendent.

Key Takeaway

Superintendents are more effective and healthier by not pretending to have all the answers or solutions to problems. Superintendents must be willing to grow stronger inner confidence that doesn't require added pressures of trying to have all the answers. No doubt, some of the questions asked of and problems experienced by superintendents are daunting and overwhelming, but being comfortable with their leadership allows them to move with a greater purpose, clarity, and inner calm.

Instead of worrying about having all the answers, it is better to embrace the opportunity to grow and seek help from others. Superintendents think that they must have all the answers and that that will establish confidence in their leadership. But that, in fact, is false. What happens is that people will stop coming to them for help, and their leadership will begin to be negatively impacted. Furthermore, this style of leadership does little for growing capacity within the district for future leaders. You must find the right balance between confidence and humility, which helps maintain effective leadership and healthy well-being. A healthy superintendent is more resilient even as they face the pressures of the job and the constant onslaught of stresses. Understanding and communicating that you do not have all the answers strengthens your ability to be more effective!

CHAPTER TWELVE

Don't Be So Hard on Yourself

"You can't be a self-leader if you are an enemy to yourself. Stop the hatred and love yourself."

—Israelmore Ayivor

Superintendents work around the clock most days and are never off the clock. When they go to the local supermarket, local library, coffee shop, or attend church services, they are seen as superintendents, not just another member of the community. Increasingly, the importance of a healthy work-life balance is coming to the forefront. Yet, somehow, the balance escapes superintendents.

At the end of the day, superintendents are too hard on themselves. Superintendents have always had the burden of the community on their shoulders, but with the global health pandemic, the burden has only multiplied and metastasized. The decisions superintendents make often result in two groups forming: those who support the decision and those who are opposed. As of late, those opposed to decisions have become more vocal in their communities, only adding to the pressures and stresses of the job.

Superintendents already had a big target on their chest due to fiscal responsibility, high-stakes testing, community support, COVID-19 protocols, Critical Race Theory (CRT), social justice, and equity, which has only made the target larger. Though they have little to no control of the community climate, they nonetheless try to lead even in the most precarious situations.

Superintendents must realize that no leader is perfect. On top of the added expectations placed on superintendents by community and government leaders, they, in fact, put extra expectations on themselves. Many superintendents live in the absolute range. For instance, superintendents may have a goal of 100 percent of students graduating in four years. Though admirable, nothing is ever 100 percent certain. Superintendents must be realistic in goal development, while still having high expectations for themselves and others.

When leaders operate in certainties, they only add to the possibilities of failure. Not being hard on themselves is not about lowering expectations or lessening the accountability that comes with the superintendency. There can still be lofty expectations and accountability, while also realistically serving as superintendent. It's natural for a leader to reflect on their decisions, to identify what worked and what didn't for future insight down the road when other decisions will be made.

Too many leaders constantly second guess their decisions, become fixated on poor decisions, and rarely compliment themselves on positive decisions. There must be a balance to maintain emotional, mental, and physical health. Decisions can eat away at a superintendent's health quickly and invisibly damage it for the long term. Superintendents, like everyone else, only have a few opportunities to make course corrections to repair their health.

Superintendents have this mindset or belief that they must make perfect decisions all the time and work inhuman hours. There is work ethic, and then there is overwork. Working tirelessly around the clock at the end of the day does not make a person a better leader. In fact, in time, the leader loses effectiveness because of poor emotional, mental, and physical health. Members of the local board of education want and need a superintendent with longevity, and this goal is compromised when superintendents continue to be hard on themselves, work around the clock, and rarely let loose and focus on their health.

The job can easily consume a person's life. Therefore, leaders must be careful. Superintendents, like other leaders, take failure personally. Taking responsibility for something that goes wrong in the school district is one thing but internalizing the failure to the point where it impacts the leader's health is completely different. Yes, the buck stops at the superintendent's desk, but the leader must be careful not to wear the problems or become consumed by failure.

Things happen in all organizations from time to time, and leadership is stressful. The key is to recognize the current situation and keep moving forward. Superintendents can't become consumed by their problems, because the problems in turn will start consuming their daily schedules at home and at work. In certain situations, superintendents begin to question their leadership abilities, which only increases stress, anxiety, self-doubt, and depression, which are crippling to a person's health.

Many superintendents acknowledge that many of the situations that are consuming are minuscule in importance, but just take a lot of time and can continue to be nagging, annoying, and time-consuming. Superintendents must be able to recognize these situations and quickly address them and keep moving. The longer the problems linger, the more superintendents will be susceptible to facing the problems and in turn begin to suffer emotionally, mentally, and physically.

Practical Strategies

1. *Reflect on decisions, but don't allow yourself to be consumed by the decision.* Superintendents must make decisions and be confident in their decisions. Too often, superintendents, like other leaders, continue to second guess their decisions. Doing so only invites lingering emotional, social, and physical health issues and stress. Be confident in the decision you make—mistakes happen, but don't continue to second guess yourself or dwell on the decision that you make.

2. *Recognize the importance of maintaining a healthy work-life balance.* No one says that the job of being superintendent must be consuming and detrimental to one's overall health. Problems can't last forever, and the superintendent can't control everything. Problems will happen, but it is important that the superintendent works to address the problems or failures that happen in the district quickly and not allow them to linger. Lingering problems only invite you to be consumed, which then begins to negatively impact your overall health and well-being.

3. *Delegate the decision-making process when you can.* Superintendents don't have to be involved in every decision. A superintendent is not effective if they are not focused on building the leadership capacity within the organization. Delegating helps superintendents to stay sharp and present each day, as they can maintain a healthy work-life balance. Furthermore, one of the most important responsibilities of a superintendent is to grow leadership capacity in the district. Nothing is more effective at growing capacity than involving others in the decision-making process and delegating authority to make decisions.

Voices from the Field

Everything Can't Go Right, 100 Percent of the Time

Bill Langley is a forty-four-year-old in his fourth year as superintendent of a school district in the Northwest. Like many superintendents, he takes things personally when something doesn't go as planned. Even when he was a teacher and principal, he always blamed himself when student achievement wasn't at the level he expected, or the graduation rate wasn't as high it could have been.

Many of his colleagues say that Bill tries to micromanage too many things and that that is why he always feels exhausted. His wife keeps telling him that if he continues to dwell on failures, the number of successes will begin to decline. He gets himself all worked up, starts questioning decisions that he made, and immediately begins to try to figure out solutions, without involving others.

Mr. Langley always felt that as a leader he was responsible for what occurred in the district. According to him, it is his responsibility to establish expectations and make sure that the district meets those expectations. Leadership requires a vision, and he works each day to make sure that everyone is working toward the same goals. Therefore, when those goals are not met, of course, he takes responsibility. That is who he is. He is repeatedly telling his colleagues, the board, and the community, he will own all failures and share all successes in the district.

When it comes to the job, Bill is extremely hard on himself. He reflects daily and makes himself sick when it comes to problems that arise, setbacks that develop, and failures in the district. He takes his job home with him, working late into the night. He still does this to this day, even though he had to visit the local emergency room because of a panic attack and irregular heartbeat. He didn't know what was happening, he couldn't catch his breath, felt anxious, and his left hand had a visible shake to it.

Sadly, he is still doing a lot of the things that he did prior to the visit to the emergency room. Bill has improved some, but he still feels as if he is responsible for everything, and people are depending on him every day to lead. Though he has cut back on work hours, he still can't let go of his district's problems and feels responsible for setbacks and failures. Now in his fourth year as a superintendent, he wonders if he will be mentally and physically capable of being a superintendent for the remainder of the school year.

Reflecting on his short tenure as a superintendent, he wishes he would have done things differently from the start. Bill should have done things differently during his time in the classroom through the principalship as well. In his mind, he mistakenly concluded that working hard, working long hours, and owning issues showed dedication. He didn't realize this level of dedication would lead to serious health issues for him as he grew older.

Mr. Langley, like many, fell into a trap that catches so many superintendents, especially new superintendents. In his mind, if he doesn't work long hours or is absent, he feels he is letting students, teachers, and principals down. He must be the one who is never absent, who accepts responsibility, and who never panics or looks nervous. All of which may sound good but, in fact, is not good for Bill's health.

In fact, it is detrimental to his health and every other superintendent who feels the same way. Bill works at getting better each day, that is, he works to not be so hard on himself. It's hard, especially as a superintendent, when people expect the chief to lead by example, have high expectations, and have the solutions to all the problems. Bill, like other superintendents, must applaud "his effort" more and blame himself less when something goes wrong.

Key Takeaway

Superintendents must reflect on why they wanted to be a superintendent. The desire and excitement about becoming the superintendent are often real until they begin to experience the demands of the job. The superintendency is a demanding job in any school district. The key for superintendents is to make sure that they are not so hard on themselves when mishaps occur, problems arise, setbacks happen, and failures ensue.

Superintendents must recognize they can't always be everywhere. Things are going to happen that are not part of the plan. That doesn't mean that they are a bad or ineffective leader, just that things happen, even in high-performing school districts. The job of the superintendent is hard and will continue to require a lot from each person in the chair. That does not mean that superintendents must compromise their health or well-being.

Furthermore, they should not compromise their personal lives or professional careers. Superintendents must realize that they have one of the best jobs in the world. They must learn how to roll with the punches but not become consumed by problems, setbacks, or failures, which will happen from time to time. The job of superintendent only requires that one establishes a culture of accountability. That does not mean that one should hold themself accountable for everything that goes wrong in the district. You can't continue to be so hard on yourself if you expect to have a long tenure or a healthy post-superintendency.

CHAPTER THIRTEEN
Don't Sweat the Small Stuff

"Don't sweat the small stuff . . . and it's all small."

—Richard Carlson

Superintendents are faced with countless questions, requests, and needs of assistance from students, teachers, staff, parents and guardians, and the community. The daily calendar of a superintendent is often filled from early morning to late into the evening. The schedule is overwhelming to the novice or veteran leader, which is why so many superintendents are retiring or leaving the profession—they can't keep up with the pace.

No matter how healthy the superintendent is, daily schedules with no downtime, no breaks, or without prioritization of importance are destined to create exhaustion and eventual burnout if something doesn't change. Everyone believes that everything should rise to the level of the superintendent, from classroom discipline, athletics, test scores, budget concerns, transportation, and so on. The list extends far beyond eyesight.

Though it is true that at the end of the day the buck stops with the superintendent, that does not mean that superintendents must have an answer to every question or solution to every problem. The decisions and concerns are too many for one person. Furthermore, everything does not require the intervention or decision of the superintendent. Leaders view trivial things as small, but they forget that even the smallest things can have a negative impact on their health if done regularly.

To maintain some semblance of sanity in their daily schedules, superintendents must prioritize their time and choose the importance of things that arrive at their desks for guidance and solutions. It is important from a mental health standpoint to have a concise and communicated organizational structure, identifying points of contact for specific areas. There is only one superintendent, and there is no way they can always be everywhere.

Likewise, there is no need for the superintendent to be responsible for answering every question and producing a solution to every problem. To find balance, the superintendent must address only important things that need a decision. They cannot sweat the small stuff; there isn't enough time in the day. Though shared decision-making is a necessity, delegation of authority to those in the organizational structure with the position to make decisions, only working with the superintendent recognizes not only how it is important for the organization and growing capacity with the organization, but it is also important to their well-being.

When decisions need to be made, by delegating the small stuff, the superintendent will be more mentally and physically fit to make the right decision. Trying to tackle every decision in the organization has a negative consequence on the overall effectiveness of their leadership, health, and well-being. Undoubtedly, the superintendent must be involved in certain decisions but not every decision.

Decisions require a certain level of energy from the leader. If the superintendent is involved in micromanaging every decision in the organization, no matter the size of the decision, at some point the leader begins to use more energy than the body can replenish daily. Therefore, many superintendents acknowledge that by the end of the day they are completely exhausted and can't make another decision. If this is how a superintendent feels every day, there is no way they are leading effectively. They may be leading by certain definitions, but let's face it, leadership does not result in mental and physical exhaustion. Yet, most superintendents do this every day. It is simply not sustainable.

Every leader will face roadblocks, obstacles, setbacks, and failures at some point in their career, as they all are part of the job of being a leader. Some leaders can endure, while others struggle with facing any obstacle. It is not that they give up, but the roadblocks, obstacles, and setbacks directly impact the leader's health. Many leaders, when they face a struggle, only increase their output, work longer hours, and jeopardize their own health and well-being, as if their effort is the reason for the obstacle or setback, no matter what they are facing.

Obstacles, setbacks, problems, and failures are stressful by nature. Leaders begin to question their own abilities, if they could have done something differently, or if they are equipped to overcome the trial and help others move forward. Some superintendents will become so obsessed with obstacles, setbacks, problems, and failures that it consumes them. They work themselves into a tizzy, only leading to increased stress and anxiety levels.

Keep in mind, medical researchers are clear that stress is deadly, especially for a prolonged period. Our bodies are not designed to endure prolonged periods of stress. Superintendents face so many things each day, their stress levels are automatically higher than most. When combined with obstacles, setbacks, problems, and failures, their stress levels drastically rise, which, if it goes unchecked, can negatively and permanently impact the superintendent's health.

Superintendents must come to grips with the fact that, yes, obstacles and problems are most assuredly going to happen, but they must not allow them to consume their lives. Obsession with an obstacle or problem does not lead to solutions, only stress, burnout, and even more obstacles and problems. Instead of becoming consumed by obstacles and problems to the point they feel exhausted, stressed, or depressed, they must let them go. This does not mean that superintendents must simply overlook them. They still need to address them, but not alone, and never to the point that their health and well-being are compromised.

At the end of the day, the superintendent must make the decision about what is big and what is small. Sometimes it is a difficult decision, but it is one that must be made not only for the health of the organization but also for their own health. Daily exhaustion and eventual burnout do nothing for the effectiveness of the organization or the superintendency but can lead to long-term health issues such as hypertension, chronic stress-related illnesses, a permanently weakened immune system, mental conditions, and eventual death. The decision the superintendent must always be involved in is the decision to prioritize their health, as no one can make this decision for them. When a superintendent looks through the lens of life, everything else seems to become small.

Practical Strategies

1. *Make a comparison.* Look through the lens of big and small. For example, solving a budget deficit is a bigger issue than choosing what is on the school lunch menu. Superintendents must weigh the decision to determine if they need to be involved or whether they can delegate to others. You can weigh the importance of the decision and determine the best path forward. Though you are the superintendent, that doesn't

mean you cannot involve others in the decision-making process or delegate the responsibility to someone else.

2. *Recognize your stressors.* No leader can make an effective decision when stressed to the limit. They are not thinking clearly. Those small decisions may seem harmless, but they require exertion of brainpower and physical energy. If a superintendent is involved in every small decision, though small, they will eventually add up to the level of a big decision. You can't allow your day to be consumed by small decisions, like determining lunch menu items, if you expect to remain sane on the job.

3. *Don't be consumed by setbacks, obstacles, and failures.* Every superintendent will face obstacles, setbacks, and failures at some point. The key for superintendents is to address them but not to allow themselves to become consumed by them. You must not dwell on them but instead address them and keep moving. There are events that need the superintendent's attention, but nothing that should make you lose focus on the job or deprioritize your own health.

4. *Schedule breaks for yourself.* Superintendents must give or create opportunities throughout the workday to take a break and disconnect from their phones, texts, emails, memos, and social media. Finding fifteen to twenty minutes each day to disconnect and take a break is transformative for your mental and physical health and well-being. Breaks allow you to refocus and make better decisions. Furthermore, breaks allow a chance for you to breathe, which is helpful, especially on stressful days.

5. *Be protective of your daily schedule.* No matter if superintendents schedule their appointments or their assistant handles their calendar, nothing goes on the schedule that doesn't need to be there. To prioritize big or trivial things requires superintendents to prioritize their schedules. They need to ask themselves whether the event, meeting, or discussion is worth putting on their schedule. Could someone else handle it? You will be surprised how massive things become small when they are prioritized on your calendars.

Voices from the Field

The Pain Associated with Stress

Dr. Rebekah Tomlison is a forty-five-year-old, sixth-year superintendent of a suburban school district on the West Coast. One of her favorite quotes is at the top of this chapter, "Don't sweat the small stuff . . . and it's all small," by Richard Carlson. She has the quote hanging on her wall in her office. Even as she has it hanging on her wall, she tells her colleagues that she contin-ues to struggle with identifying what is small and what is big in her role as a superintendent. She tends to want to classify everything as major and is involved in every decision.

Rebekah has become so consumed by decisions that she regularly becomes exhausted. She doesn't get hung up on setbacks, but she does allow herself to be consumed with making decisions. She works to the point of exhaustion and then questions why she feels bad, becomes sick, or a body part is sore or aching. It is who she is, and she works every day trying to overcome this work routine. Though she still struggles with taking on too much, she has made major improvements because of an episode she had near the end of the school year a couple of years ago.

The school year was particularly difficult. The district had to make bud-get cuts the year before, and projections showed that it would have to make additional budget cuts the next school year. Class sizes increased as the dis-trict reduced staff to address declining revenues and then limited purchases, field trips, and other supports that students, teachers, and staff had become accustomed to having in previous school years.

Dr. Tomlison worked closely with members of the board of education and kept them up to speed with what was occurring and the reasons behind decreasing revenues. Any time a superintendent must make decisions about the budget, it is difficult, as the budget impacts everything in the school district. Rebekah spent a lot of hours going through the budget line by line.

Furthermore, she was involved in many meetings over many months. Rebekah was working seven days a week, even convening budget meetings on the weekend with the finance officer and district team members. She was working to the point of exhaustion and dragging members of her leadership team along with her. Her team was concerned for Rebekah and their own health, as eighty-plus hours per week became the norm for several months.

It was Rebekah's responsibility to present to the board a recommenda-tion about the budget cuts. No one else could do it. At some point the week before the board meeting and about ten days before graduation, she started to notice a soreness in her left knee and her toes on her left foot. She thought she had sprained her knee and foot somehow, but she hadn't been physically active for a while. Steadily, the soreness turned to pain. After a couple of days of increasing pain in both her knee and toes, she couldn't walk without assistance.

Rebekah's secretary scheduled an appointment with her physician for later that morning. By the time 11:00 a.m. rolled around, she was experienc-ing excruciating pain and had removed her left shoe. One of the assistant superintendents drove her to her appointment as she could not concentrate on driving due to the pain. When she got to the physician's office, she had to use a wheelchair to enter the office.

When the doctor finally came into the room, he examined Rebekah's foot and quickly diagnosed her with gout. Gout is a form of inflammatory arthritis that can lead to mild or excruciating pain. When the doctor said gout, she said, "Gout? But I don't eat a lot of red meat, tomatoes, all the things that you see on television as causes of gout." She assumed like many it was something she was eating that caused her setback, but there is more to the story.

What the doctor said next struck her totally by surprise. He knew Rebekah was superintendent and asked if she had been under a lot of stress lately. The doctor said that gout can also be caused by stress, not necessarily by diet. She told her doctor that the past three weeks had been exceedingly difficult and stressful, causing her to work more than normal. Her physician said that her body had finally caught up with her because of the stress.

The doctor gave her some advice that goes through my head every time I get involved in a decision. Rebekah's physician told her that at some point, she needed to let things go and let things play out and stop trying to control everything. He said he has no doubt that she was a good superintendent, but she didn't need to agonize over every decision. Plus, he recommended that she stop working so many hours. Rebekah, especially during stressful weeks, needs time to separate from the job and allow her mind and body to rejuvenate. She couldn't keep placing this amount of stress on herself.

Dr. Tomlison's physician gave her some medication that helped, but he wrote a prescription and handed it to her. It said, "Don't sweat the small stuff and everything is small." She mentioned that she had this quote hanging in her office. When she got to her office, she taped her prescription note to her desk so that she could see it when she felt stressed or was working too much. She now tries to delegate as much as possible, but she still finds herself gravitating to decision-making. Every time she gets tied up in decisions, her staff now reminds her to look at the prescription card and do what the doctor said . . . Don't sweat the small stuff!

Key Takeaway

Like the doctor says, "Don't sweat the small stuff." You must let go sometimes and not dwell on decisions, obstacles, setbacks, or failures. There is nothing positive that comes from dwelling on the past. Superintendents must continue to move forward so that the district can move forward. This starts with superintendents recognizing the big and small decisions that must be made. Furthermore, superintendents should realize that they do not need to be involved in every decision. Informed? Yes. Kept abreast of the decision? Yes. But they do not necessarily need to be an integral part of the decision-making process.

As the superintendency continues to transform, with the call and need for more collaboration with others in the district, hopefully, superintendents will not have to be so involved. This is not to suggest that superintendents can stay in their office and not know what is going on in the district. It just means that they need to step back some and allow others to be involved in the decision-making process.

Superintendents will be challenged with deciding what is big and small. A rule of thumb is to evaluate who the decision will impact and what is the long-term effect of the decision being made. If superintendents can slow down to evaluate each obstacle, problem, decision, setback, and failure, they will not only be able to determine their involvement, but also continue to move forward with less stress and more energy!

CHAPTER FOURTEEN

Discover Your Release

"It's not the load that breaks you down, it's the way you carry the load."
—Lou Holtz

An around-the-clock schedule, for 365 days each year, is not sustainable for the long term. If by chance a superintendent can pull off working around the clock for years, eventually it catches up with their health. Honestly, burnout or exhaustion has long-lasting effects on the person that sometimes is irreparable. The body and mind are amazingly resilient; however, eventually, a person can get to a point that no amount of therapy or medication can help.

No superintendent is expected to work to the point of exhaustion. Yet, hundreds, if not thousands, work to the point of exhaustion each day across the nation. These same superintendents are speeding toward a brick wall called reality. Eventually, a person's health always catches up with them. The mind and body are built for struggles and hardship but not repeated trauma.

Let's be clear, constant day in and day out exhaustion is a form of trauma that leads to serious medical conditions that end a superintendency. It is humanly impossible and irresponsible to work to the point of exhaustion each day when there are easier and healthier ways to lead. Highly effective superintendents prioritize their schedules. They work hard each day and give the job 100 percent each day, but they also make their own health a priority.

They understand that their health is critical to their role as a leader. Without their health and well-being, high-performing leaders recognize that their tenure is destined to be short and not overly successful. But more importantly, they have come to realize how important it is to have release mechanisms when the job becomes too stressful or when the job becomes taxing on their time each day.

One of the most successful ways to lower stress and rejuvenate the body and mind is to have a release strategy. There are several release strategies that are available to any leader, but the key is the leader and choosing the right release for them. What may work for one leader may not work for another. Also, a leader may use a variety of release strategies, instead of choosing just one. From walking, sitting in total silence, taking the day off, exercising, reading, journaling, or listening to music, the leader must identify what works best for them.

Release requires just as much dedication as the job of the superintendent itself. If a leader half commits to their release, they will only get half of the reward. As superintendents prioritize their job professionally, they must also prioritize their release strategies for themselves personally. Surprisingly, those superintendents who practice release strategies regularly are more effective and healthier, as opposed to those superintendents who think wasting time away from the job, even spending five minutes, makes them less effective.

A healthy well-being is a prerequisite to leadership effectiveness. Superintendents who are not healthy are not able to commit 100 percent to the job because they are constantly overcome by exhaustion or other health issues. In other words, superintendents prioritizing their health and finding time to have a release maximizes the time that they can spend focused on the job. Superintendents underestimate, like others, the power of having a release.

Superintendents taking time for themselves and using personalized release strategies may seem to them that they are not putting forth 100 percent into the job. They also may feel bad taking time for themselves, while others are working nonstop. The beauty is that the more the leader prioritizes health and well-being it trickles down to others. It is amazing how health, well-being, and organizational culture are all connected. To have a healthy organizational culture, the leader must be healthy, as well as the employees. At the end of the day, superintendents want a positive, high-energy, and healthy culture, which starts with the superintendent modeling the way for others.

As a profession, superintendents must understand that working longer hours and more days does not equate to effectiveness, in fact, exactly the opposite. If a superintendent fails to give themselves a break throughout the day and find time for themselves, they can't fully commit to the job and can't be there for others like they could if they were not so exhausted, fatigued, and tired. The superintendency demands a lot from each leader and so does the leader's health and well-being. Prioritizing health and well-being does not take time from the job. It actually adds more opportunities to commit to the job and be more present, leading to improved effectiveness without jeopardizing overall health and well-being.

Practical Strategies

1. *Identify and recognize when you become stressed.* Superintendents must listen to and observe what is happening to the mind, body, and soul. Once they become stressed or approach exhaustion, they must utilize the strategies that work for them to lower their stress. Your health and well-being are uniquely individual; therefore, your release must be tailored to your needs. You must identify and utilize the releases that work for you, whether that is exercising, journaling, or listening to music.

2. *Accept that you too are human.* Superintendents don't need to feel embarrassed or think of themselves as weak if they become stressed, exhausted, or more importantly, if they must take time for themselves. As superintendents prioritize their health, they will become better positioned to help others and to commit to the superintendency more effectively. There is nothing shameful or weak about prioritizing your health. Superintendents, like other leaders, are not invincible.

3. *Schedule a time during the day to take a break.* If superintendents are concerned that they won't recognize when they are approaching their limit or they can't recognize when they are stressed, then they should schedule time each day to take a break. Again, fifteen to twenty minutes each day can be transformative for a leader's effectiveness and health. At the end of the day, the fifteen to twenty minutes you spend on yourself will not take away from your duties or effectiveness as superintendent. In fact, you will find your day more rewarding and have an overall sense of accomplishment. More importantly, you will feel healthier and not exhausted. Therefore, you can spend more quality time after work with friends and family, which also helps your overall health and well-being.

Voices from the Field

Family Can Fix All Problems

Robert Patterson is a forty-two-year-old male in his third year as superintendent of a suburban school district in the Northeast. As a third-year superintendent, he has experienced several situations and scenarios in a brief time in the district. He is regularly invited to speak to aspiring superintendents and present at conferences.

Over Robert's tenure as superintendent, it has taken some time to find his release. Like many superintendents, he struggles with the work-life balance. Finding the right path to separate home and the office is difficult and does not occur overnight. Typically, when superintendents do find the right balance, it is out of necessity due to a health issue, exhaustion, or personal reasons.

Robert often tells aspiring superintendents that his life doesn't revolve around his role as superintendent, or, at least, he tries to make sure that it doesn't. He has a wife and a twelve-year-old son who is in middle school, and they like to do things as a family. He married his college sweetheart and has been blessed in so many ways. Both he and his wife are educators. She is a first-grade teacher in a neighboring school district, and she is a rockstar. If social media posts from her student's parents are an indication of the caliber of teacher she is, she is exemplary, as the comments are always complimentary of her.

Robert loves his family and enjoys being a superintendent. As a family, the Pattersons do so many things together that he can't imagine not spending time with them both. His son is active in sports at school, playing a sport every season. Robert enjoys going to his son's home and away games, though he sometimes must miss away games due to district meetings. But he makes certain that he only misses a few each season, as he wants to be involved and show his support. Plus, it gives him and his wife an opportunity to spend time together.

Mr. Patterson considers himself healthy and works out regularly at home. He and his wife will take walks together in the neighborhood in the evening and on the weekends. He plays sports with his son and his friends after work if he gets home early enough, but especially on weekends. Robert hates going home and just sitting. He has never been a huge fan of sitting and wants to keep moving. His mind never stops, and he is always moving in an effective way, not to the point of exhaustion.

How effective is Mr. Patterson at being a superintendent? How can he be an effective superintendent if he is spending so much time with his family?

Frequent questions for many. Working with fellow superintendents in his regional co-op, he hears stories of superintendents spending fifty-plus hours at work, not including working at home in the evening to get everything accomplished. His colleagues talk about how tired they are, how their bodies hurt, or how much weight they have gained. Some of them even talk about how their marriage is on the rocks because they are rarely home.

When Robert became superintendent, because of his wife and son, he swore that he would not become a victim of the job. From the beginning, he controlled his own schedule and made certain that family time was scheduled, as it should be. This doesn't mean that he didn't get home late some nights each week, but most evenings and weekends he spent with his family doing family things. His job is incredibly important to him, but his family is more important. Members of the board of education seem not to have a problem with how he is leading, as he has always been upfront with them about how important his family is to him.

So, what is Robert's release? The answer is that he enjoys spending time with his family. He has had some rough days with several meetings and making tough decisions. The job sometimes wears him down. But when he arrives home and can sit down to have dinner with his wife and son, he is reinvigorated. Talking about their day and what they are going to do on the weekend helps the stress subside. Evenings, whether at home or at one of his son's games, help Robert to re-center on his health and why he must remain healthy so that he can spend more time with his family.

Many superintendents who are reading this have not yet found their release. Their release may not be their family; it may be exercise, crafting, reading, or listening to music. Superintendents are encouraged to find a release to help cope with the many stresses of the job. For a third-year superintendent, Robert knows without his release, he would also be talking about exhaustion and being overwhelmed. The superintendency is hard, but that doesn't mean it can't be healthy or has to be counterproductive to the leader's health. Robert made a promise to himself and his family that if the job became too much to the point he started missing family time, he would quit.

Key Takeaway

A release does not have to be sophisticated or expensive. In fact, the best release for leaders is simple and free. A superintendent's release may be staring at them in the face, but they are too busy to see it. You must think about what you enjoy doing the most. You may enjoy crafting, journaling, building things, reading, listening to music, spending time with friends, or exercising.

No matter what it is, use it as a release. The key thing to remember about a release is that it's utilized regularly, not sporadically.

If a superintendent has had a tough day or week, they need to make time to release their stress and anxiety. Again, their release doesn't have to take up a lot of time, just fifteen to twenty minutes, but nothing says it can't be longer if needed. There is nothing wrong with prioritizing your health and well-being. If you can find time to do something that you enjoy that is not connected to the job, you will be surprised how much better you will be as a superintendent. You can only take so much. But by knowing your release, you can find a healthier work-life balance.

CHAPTER FIFTEEN
Listen to What Your Body Is Telling You

"Your body is like the quiet talker with the most important thing to say."
—Marissa Vicario

Too many people, including school superintendents, only pay attention to their health when it's too late. As humans, we are equipped with an early warning system, which, if we listen closely and pay attention to it, will tell us when to slow down and take a break. Unfortunately, too many superintendents hear, feel, and see the early signs of exhaustion, burnout, and health impairments, yet they continue to push forward.

When leaders see bags under their eyes, changing skin colors, new body or joint aches, regular headaches, shortness of breath, or constant feelings of fatigue, often their body is telling them it's time to slow down. Superintendents do not have unlimited fuel or energy. Likewise, superintendents are not expected to risk their health just for the job, though we see obituaries daily of current superintendents who passed away while still a superintendent. This doesn't include superintendents who pass away shortly after retirement. The correlation is the job—poor dieting, less exercise, more stress, and less time away from the job. All are prerequisites for burnout, fatigue, hypertension, and shorter life spans.

Though death may seem like an exaggeration, the facts don't lie. Superintendents are so shackled to their jobs, with little or no separation between home and work, they are working themselves out of a job and into the grave. Even if by chance superintendents can retire, their quality and length of life are negatively impacted. Superintendents have dedicated their entire career to helping others, only to retire with little to show for it, except poor health.

Again, the body is sending signals, if superintendents will only slow down, listen, and pay attention to the messages. These messages will help protect against personal harm. Taking five to ten minutes each day, before work, during the day, and after work, to check themselves mentally, emotionally, and physically can lead to surprising and positive outcomes for superintendents. Again, people at some point will make health and well-being a priority, but too often, it's too late to correct the health spiral to long-term and permanent severe health conditions and even death. Surely, superintendents can afford to take twenty minutes each day to check on their health. What could be more important than their own health?

Listening to our bodies is not an easy thing to do—for anyone, including superintendents—especially when the job consumes most of their lives. Listening to your body is not a one-time thing. We only listen when we have reached the point of exhaustion, but it may be too late to correct the path. Superintendents should be monitoring what their bodies are telling them each day, Monday through Sunday. When they begin to listen to their bodies, it is amazing what people will find out about themselves and how much better they feel about themselves. Everything that could happen to our health, our bodies are equipped to send warning signals about.

Hindsight is always twenty-twenty, but right now, superintendents need to develop a twenty-twenty vision when it comes to their health and well-being. There are so many red flags that if superintendents will slow down and pay attention, they can bypass burnout, exhaustion, serious health concerns, and even death. The superintendency is nothing to take lightly, nor is your health and well-being. You only have one body, and right now it may be telling you to slow down, work smarter, not harder, and make time for yourself to rejuvenate and breathe. Just listen to your body. It has something important to tell you, always, before it's too late. Eventually, we all must make our health a priority, either as a preventative strategy or a reaction, due to serious health concerns and issues.

Practical Strategies

1. *Time management is essential to hearing and seeing signals.* You must give yourself breaks throughout the day where you are alone to catch your breath and to clear your mind. This will allow you to reflect and allow your body to recover from the stresses of the job. Don't fool yourself,

the superintendency is stressful and can have a lasting negative consequence for your body if left unattended or disregarded.

2. *Trust your body's signals.* Early warning signs usually come in the form of new sporadic headaches, joint pains, dizziness, loss of sleep, and stomach pains. In severe cases, trouble breathing or chest pains are urgent signals. These are symptoms that you should not allow to go unchecked. This is the time to speak with a physician, take a break, disconnect, and disengage from work for a little while.

3. *Dismount and disengage.* Though you may think you can continue to ride the mechanical bull that is the superintendency forever, at some point your body will make you dismount if you don't heed the warning signs. Sometimes you must let go and disengage from the job. This doesn't mean leaving work early and then returning to the same daily grind the very next day. Yes, take afternoons off when you need to, but to dismount and disengage you need to step away from the job for days, weeks, or an extended period of time. There is never a good time to be away from the job, but if your heart, soul, body, and mind need a break, they need a break. If they go unreplenished, irreparable harm is not far away.

4. *Slow down to speed up.* Superintendents, to be effective, do not need to speed up, work around the clock, and always be available for the job. The best strategy is to slow down so that you can become a more effective, healthier leader. Working around the clock to the point of exhaustion and sacrificing sleep for last-minute deadlines is not a sustainable strategy and does not equate to effective leadership. Speed sometimes outpaces the body, which delays warning signals. By slowing down, your body can communicate its needs better.

Voices from the Field

Slow Down and Listen

Marisa Sanchez is a fifty-seven-year-old female who has served as superintendent for the past five years in a district located in the Southwest. She is currently in her fifth year as a superintendent and she has failed miserably in paying attention to her health and well-being, as Marisa tells her superintendent friends.

Each week, by the time she makes it to Friday, she is completely exhausted. She can barely move, and most weekends she lies on the couch or bed and stays home if she doesn't have a school or community event or commitment.

Before becoming superintendent, Marisa participated in annual marathons, which she enjoyed immensely, as she would run with her lifelong friends since elementary school.

Prior to becoming a superintendent, she considered herself healthy, rarely ever having to go to the doctor. She was so healthy, she rarely had a cold during the winter months. She watched what she ate and made sure that she got plenty of sleep, even as a middle school principal. When Ms. Sanchez became superintendent, her goal was to keep running marathons and keep doing all the other things that helped her to remain healthy.

The first year was good but not great in terms of her dedication to her health. She ran a marathon; however, it was challenging for her. Typically, her practice leading up to a marathon consisted of running three to four times each week while consuming water, watching her diet, and getting plenty of rest and sleep. For this marathon during her first year as superintendent, Marisa practiced, but it was sporadic, and she could never get a running routine like she needed and enjoyed in the past.

She gained five pounds, which may seem not terrible to many but for a runner can have an enormous impact. Plus, she was working seven days a week, never giving her body rest, and her sleep routine changed from an average of seven hours per night before becoming a superintendent to only four hours as a superintendent. A month after she finished the marathon during her first year as superintendent, she noticed that she was always sore and achy.

She had tension in her neck, and she could never stretch the soreness out of her neck or body. As a runner, she knew how to stretch and always made it a priority before and after she finished running. This soreness, especially around her neck, caught her off guard, but at first, she didn't think too much about it. After three weeks of constant tension in her neck, which was becoming increasingly painful and aggravating, she went to a chiropractor even though she didn't want to.

The chiropractor worked and massaged her neck, which helped, and that night she was finally able to sleep. The next day by noon, the tension was back and more painful. That caused Marisa to go to the emergency room because she was afraid that she might have been experiencing a stroke, due to the pain she was experiencing in her neck. Marisa was hooked up to every type of machine, and the emergency room nurses were treating her as if she was having a stroke, but all the tests came back as normal.

After spending half the day in the emergency room, the attending physician sent her home with a muscle relaxer, told her to take a couple of days off, and told her if the problems persist that she needed to see her regular physician. The next day at work, Mrs. Sanchez decided against taking sick leave or slowing down. She showed up to work early trying to make up for the lost time the day before and trying to get ahead.

Her neck felt fine, and she thought it was just something minor. By Friday evening, her neck pain had returned, and the left side of her face felt numb. Her husband called 911, and she was rushed to the hospital where she again was plugged into every machine for tests. On Friday, May 11, she suffered a mild stroke. The pain was a small blood clot in her neck that was also causing the numbness in her face according to the doctors.

In this instance, Marisa's body was telling her something was wrong, and the added stress of the job only compounded the issues. Her body was in shock after being healthy for years, after a year of being a superintendent and not taking care of herself. Her body wasn't accustomed to this level of stress, poor diet, lack of sleep, and lack of exercise. It took several days before the feeling returned to the left side of her face, but this time she took not days but weeks off.

For a person who was healthy before the superintendency and now needs to pay close attention to her body, Marisa struggles with allowing herself to get into this shape. But something good did come from the stroke, as she is now back running three times per week, watching what she eats, and making sure that she gets enough sleep at night. It is easy for superintendents to get lost in their job and forget about their health.

So far, no neck pain or other symptoms have returned. Marisa's body was telling her to slow down, and she learned the hard way. She has cut back on her hours at work, delegated to others, but more importantly, she is back running three times per week with her friends. Throughout this ordeal, one positive thing emerged. As a result of listening to what her body was telling her and again prioritizing her health, she often tells colleagues that she believes that she is a better superintendent for focusing on herself.

Key Takeaway

That new headache, knee pain, chronic pain in your stomach, chest pain, or dizziness is your body telling you that something needs to change quickly. If you are moving at lightning speed and overlook these signals your body is sending you, beware, there is trouble on the horizon. Your body is a sophisticated machine that sends us signals each day about a variety of things, including our health. These signals should not be overlooked.

Superintendents become so focused on the job that a lot of times they misinterpret the signals or completely miss the signals. These signals are not optional and must be addressed as soon as possible. The body sends these signals as a warning, and in the case of superintendents, tells them to find time to focus on their health and well-being. Though the body is a sophisticated machine, it is not injury-proof, especially if it is not a priority. Time is always an issue, but eventually, if not prioritized, our body will make superintendents make time for their health if it's not too late.

CHAPTER SIXTEEN
Embrace Personal Accountability

"It's only when you take responsibility for your life, that you discover
how powerful you truly are!"

—Allanah Hunt

Accountability and education are synonymous. In fact, today's education is
driven by accountability in that it is based on student test scores. Surprisingly, however, most superintendents struggle with personal accountability.
They work long hours, give up their personal lives, and put their health and
well-being on the backburner each day. Superintendents are focused on
everything and everyone else, often only thinking about themselves when
it's too late.

Personal accountability, in today's school districts, is needed, specifically
by superintendents. This isn't about the superintendent owning a district-
level decision or a mistake that occurred but taking responsibility for their
own health. This may include owning a decision, but in this case, it's a personal decision. Superintendents must own the outcomes of not focusing on
their health and well-being, just as much as they own budget, personnel, or
academic decisions.

There must be a change in thinking in the superintendency in which
superintendents are accountable to the public for district-related decisions
and outcomes as well as their own health and well-being. Unfortunately,
just as superintendents must lead change within schools, they must also lead
this change as well. Only superintendents can make their own health and

well-being a priority. There is no board of education, legislature, or organization that can make this important for superintendents.

Health and well-being are not things that can be "willed" by someone or into existence. Health and well-being require dedication, patience, and understanding. Superintendents can't focus on their health one day and forget about it the next. Likewise, they must practice patience, as transformation in health and well-being can never be rushed. Additionally, superintendents must understand and recognize just how important their health and well-being are to their effectiveness as leaders. A leader cannot lead if their health and well-being are compromised.

The same level of accountability that superintendents hold themselves to when it comes to achievement gaps must be transferred to their own health and well-being. If your diet isn't the best, what are you going to do about it? If you are fatigued all the time, what are you going to do about it? If you are working eighty-plus hours a week and missing time with your family, what are you going to do about it? Just as superintendents would make changes to reading strategies or programs to improve third-grade reading scores in their school district, they must make changes in their personal and professional lives.

The superintendency is short. No matter if the tenure of a superintendent lasts three years or twenty years, it is relative to a leader's health and well-being. Though the superintendent may have the best intentions, by working long hours, not taking time off, or spending time with family, the result is never positive or promising. The outcome is always detrimental to a leader, personally and professionally.

Superintendents must develop the understanding that when they prioritize their own health and well-being, they become better leaders and can better help others to focus on their own health and well-being. Personal accountability doesn't stop with solely focusing on their own health. Instead, superintendents must model the way for others. This alone should ignite the inner drive of accountability.

If the superintendent will not do it for themselves, they should at least do it for others. Though it may be difficult to believe, a superintendent's focus on health and well-being is transformative to a district's culture and the lives of the staff and students. When the leader is healthy, they work to create a healthy organizational culture and focus on the social, emotional, and physical well-being of staff and students.

To be clear, the problem facing superintendents, whether they recognize it or not, is their long-term health and well-being. Though it may not be confronting them at this exact moment in time, if they continue to work to the point of mental and physical exhaustion, their health and well-being will be damaged, in many cases permanently. Though the superintendency tomorrow may be more complicated, that doesn't mean that leaders must continue to sacrifice their own health and well-being for the job.

There is a balance, no matter the demands of the office. You can and must step away, take a breath, go for a walk, take a vacation, or go out with friends and family. Superintendents must continue to hold themselves for district-related matters. Likewise, they must begin holding themselves to the same level of accountability when it comes to their health and well-being. Don't run from holding yourself accountable for your health.

More importantly, don't feel ashamed either. When you must take fifteen minutes to breathe, or leave work early to do something with your family, or go to the gym before you go to school, be proud and confident that you are doing the right thing for the long journey that lies ahead. Make changes, prioritize, and hold yourself accountable. Don't allow yourself to overlook your health, just like you wouldn't allow third-grade reading scores to be overlooked.

Practical Strategies

1. *Prioritize your schedule.* Superintendents are extremely busy, no matter the size of the school district. But they should not be too busy to make their health and well-being a priority in the district. Superintendents control their schedules; they decide the number of meetings each day, the length of meetings, which schools they are visiting, and who they meet with daily. This same level of control must be afforded to their health and well-being. Dedicating time during the day, twenty minutes here and there throughout the day, can be transformative to your health and well-being. Health and well-being require your attention, but on the scale of everything, it doesn't need to consume a lot of your time.

2. *Trade-off events.* If a superintendent works late one evening, then the next evening, they should prioritize getting home early to have dinner with family, go to the gym, go for a walk, or all three. There must be trade-offs to establish a healthy work-life balance. You cannot work late every night and expect not to become exhausted. Trade-offs do not equate to being ineffective or failing on your responsibilities. In fact, balancing your schedule will help you to be more present and effective, and additionally, healthier.

3. *Establish goals for your health and well-being, and measure regularly.* Consider this continuous improvement for your health. Just as superintendents monitor student attendance data, reading data, graduation data, they must also monitor data pertaining to their own health and well-being. At home or at work, or both, track your work hours, your diet, exercise, minutes meditating, and other health data such as blood pressure and weight. If the data suggests problems with your health and well-being, make the necessary changes. Hold yourself accountable to make the changes in your work schedule to create a healthier work-life balance.

Voices from the Field

Own Your Health

Dr. Peter Goodwill is a thirty-seven-year-old male in his second year as a superintendent of a rural school district on the West Coast. Prior to becoming a superintendent, he was active, ran marathons, and enjoyed spending time at home with friends and family. Peter is constantly being asked by principals and other superintendents how he stays in shape. He doesn't believe in magic bullets or tricks. Since college, he has kept track of his health and well-being, sometimes at obsessive levels, but he is glad he did.

Peter is in his fifteenth year of his career, but second as a superintendent. Over the fifteen years, he may have been absent only one day, and he credits that to his focus on his health. His mentors warned him that when he became a superintendent he would totally change—physically, mentally, and emotionally. Throughout his superintendent preparation program, there was nothing about the importance of health and well-being mentioned for leaders. Nationally, research and guidance for superintendents in terms of health and well-being remains a problem.

Luckily, Dr. Goodwill went into the superintendency with his eyes wide open. He realizes that he is part of a small population of superintendents who prioritize their health over the job. He knew and understood the importance of health and well-being. If he had not been physically active and diet-conscious, he could easily have allowed the job to run away with his health. The superintendency, if one is not careful, can be overwhelming and detrimental to a person's health and well-being.

Peter recognized the importance of self-control and personal accountability. He constantly reminded himself about the dangers of the job and the potential of falling victim to bad health habits, like he knew others did. He paid attention to his health and well-being. He was working to not become exhausted, overweight, or overall unhealthy mentally, emotionally, and physically. His goal was to remain in the superintendency for the remainder of his career.

Dr. Goodwill made a concerted effort to keep his health and well-being a priority. Though he did have to make concessions, like the number of days that he would go to the gym, he still schedules gym time. Furthermore, he seldom checks email on weekends unless it's an emergency, and people know how to reach him if there is an emergency. He spends time with his wife and ten-year-old daughter on the weekends. He also makes sure that he attends all his daughter's after-school events.

Peter utilizes a strategy when he notices that his schedule is getting out of control—too many meetings during the day, spending less time in school(s), or too many after-work events. He works with his executive assistant to rearrange meetings and delegate to directors if possible. He is adamant about squeezing in time for himself throughout the day so he can decompress.

He silences his phone and does not check email or scroll through social media. Peter tries not to stay in his office, but be out in schools performing walkthroughs, talking with principals, custodians, bus drivers, teachers, and students. In other words, he kills two birds with one stone—he is in schools but moving, releasing stress, and breathing. He always has his health and well-being on his mind, even as he carries out the duties of a superintendent.

Peter doesn't blame anyone else for his health—he owns this responsibility. If the job gets out of control, that is also on him. He makes sure that he pays attention to his schedule and his health. On Sunday afternoons, he reviews his exercise journal from the previous week and tries to improve his exercises and availability to exercise for the upcoming week. This requires him to be strategic with his weekly calendar. If one day is packed and shortens his opportunity to exercise, he tries to make up the minutes lost the next day. He never goes two days without some form of exercise.

Superintendents must take responsibility for their health. They can't blame their secretaries, physicians, spouses, or the job if their health gets out of control. Superintendents must own their health. Furthermore, they must make certain that each day they do something that will help maintain tier health. Don't become a superintendent who must leave the job in five years because of health or being exhausted. Be in for the long haul! To do so, it is imperative for health to be prioritized and have it on one's schedule both at home and at work.

Key Takeaway

Superintendents must never underestimate just how much control they have over their own health and well-being. Their health is too important to delegate to others. It is incumbent upon the superintendent to emphasize and communicate the importance of health and well-being throughout the school district. A culture of well-being goes a long way in helping superintendents, but even then, superintendents are responsible for their district's culture.

Personal accountability requires a certain level of continuous improvement by superintendents. Just as superintendents track student data, they must also track their own data, to make improvements in their health and well-being. Improvements in their health and well-being will not just happen, there must be a strategic approach, prioritization of schedules, and honesty with themselves.

If a superintendent's health isn't improving, then changes need to be made, but the superintendent must not look the other way when they begin to realize their health and well-being is not in optimal condition. You must be honest with yourself (personal accountability), slow down, and prioritize your health. Just as you have high expectations for other areas of the job, have the same high expectations for your own health.

CHAPTER SEVENTEEN

You Are Only the Superintendent, Not Superhuman

"If you try to do too much, you will not achieve anything."
—Confucius

Every superintendent falls into what is called the superman or superwoman trap from time to time, especially novice leaders. Superintendents are looked to for leadership in their school districts and communities. In many times, the superintendent may be the only leader in communities, especially in rural or bush communities that exist throughout the nation. But this does not mean that leaders in more populated and urban superintendents are not looked to as leaders in their communities.

In every community, when it comes to education, teachers, staff members, parents, guardians, and members of the community look to the superintendent for leadership in a variety of areas, not solely in education. Since March 2020, due to COVID-19, social justice movements, attacks on boards of education, Critical Race Theory (CRT) discussions, the banning of certain books, and so many other things, superintendents have been looked to for leadership, yes, but also to be a community activist, peace officer, counselor, and a medical advisor. This is not an over-exaggeration of what has been placed on the superintendent's plate.

The past two years have been very tough, but even before then, superintendents have always been expected to possess superhuman traits. This expectation goes far beyond having all the answers and, sometimes, goes to the extreme. Superintendents are human just like everyone else, but in many cases, they are expected to work ridiculously unhealthy, long hours each week, never take breaks or vacation, and focus on everyone else's needs, while their needs and families are forced to the bottom of the priority list.

We must keep in mind that there are many superintendents who struggle waking up each day as their emotional, mental, and physical health and well-being are not the best, and, in some cases, dangerously not well. The superintendency can easily become out of control for any leader. Though the job starts out demanding a little more each day from the superintendent, eventually, if not monitored, it becomes out of control, and that is when everything goes out of balance, especially the superintendent's health and well-being.

Even superman and superwoman must sleep, though superintendents today believe they must always be available for the job. Superintendents who believe that they can be effective leaders with no sleep or an inadequate amount of sleep are fooling themselves and are destined to fail and, even worse, have severe health issues. No job description for any superintendent says that they must put their own health and well-being at risk, though the job continues to morph into something bigger each year, demanding more from each leader.

A superintendent's kryptonite is their health and well-being. If the superintendent is expected to possess superhuman strength and powers, they must first make sure that their health and well-being are at their peak. This requires that superintendents prioritize sleep, diet, exercise, time away from the job, and their families. But to be clear, superintendents should not be prioritizing those things just to be superhuman, but instead, to ensure a healthy emotional, mental, and physical well-being.

Don't try to be superman or superwoman. No board of education nor community expects you to jeopardize your health. Furthermore, no superintendent possesses superhuman powers or strengths. Superintendents are human, just like the members of the board, teachers, principals, parents, and members of the community. Superintendents are leaders in their communities, but to be effective and serve with longevity, they must maintain a healthy work-life balance. Just as superman prioritized his health—hence his physique—superintendents must also prioritize their health.

Practical Strategies

1. *Delegate when possible.* Superintendents do not need to be involved in every decision made in the district. Furthermore, many superintendents have learned that they do not need to be at every meeting that happens throughout the district. The best way to not be expected to be everything to everybody is to empower others to be leaders and go-to

people in the district. By doing so, you are not only protecting your health but also building leadership capacity within the district.

2. *Understand that you are not superman.* Just as important, superintendents can't be superman. Superintendents can't be everywhere and expect to get things done. Furthermore, superintendents can't be everything to everybody and be expected to be effective and to last long. Furthermore, a recipe for failure is for the superintendent to expect to be for everybody and everywhere they are needed. Priorities matter, empowering others matter, and being realistic absolutely matters.

3. *Embrace the vulnerability of being human.* Superman and superwoman would struggle to be a leader because of their vulnerabilities, which makes them unreal. Heroes are not necessarily leaders. Boards of education, parents, and communities want a leader, not necessarily a hero. Leaders learn from their shortcomings and experiences. Leaders fail, and they become stronger. Think about how many times superman or superwoman has ever failed—few, if any. However, leaders fail often, learn, and become better for it, which is precisely what school districts need. People are more likely to associate with leaders than heroes because, like them, leaders are vulnerable, and that isn't necessarily a terrible thing.

Voices from the Field

Kryptonite

Dr. Elizabeth St. Claire is a fifty-five-year-old female who has served as superintendent of a small district in the Northeast for the past ten years. Right out of the gate, she thought she possessed superhuman abilities, that is, she believed she could work around the clock, be at every meeting and event, and be there to answer all questions that may arise. She had to be the exact opposite of her predecessor, whose contract was not renewed because he was rarely in the office or in schools and rarely provided guidance in most school district matters.

Elizabeth fell victim to trying to compare herself to another superintendent. Her predecessor was known for delegating a lot. The problem was when he delegated to others, he wouldn't tell anyone, therefore blindsiding them. She was set out to prove that she was a better leader, and she worked daily, too much, to achieve this goal. What started out as a goal became an obsession that brought concerns with her health and well-being.

She wanted to be different, and she was a new superintendent with the burning fire to make a difference in the district. Elizabeth had a list of things that she wanted to accomplish in her first and second years, and she shared the list with the board of education. She started out slowly but somehow convinced herself that she could get the two-page list done in six months. At first, she was crossing items off the list every week. Keep in mind, her two-page list of priorities was full-page, front and back.

Today, Elizabeth realizes that she moved too fast for the organization and that she only exhausted herself. It got to the point, after being on the job for two months, that she ended up in the emergency room with a migraine. Prior to becoming a superintendent, she rarely experienced headaches, but what she was doing to herself each day eventually led to a migraine. This is a classic example of the job negatively impacting the leader's health.

She now experiences chronic migraines because of stress and has to take a daily prescription. What makes matters worse is that when she developed the migraines, because she put too much stress on herself, she would become stressed even more because it was debilitating to her. It was a cycle of migraines triggered by the amount of stress she was placing on herself each day.

Some days were better than others, but when she experiences a severe migraine, she isolates at home, in a guest room with no light, no noise and no cell phone, just total peace and calm. Though she thought she was a super-woman, she found her kryptonite (stress) two months into the job, and she has been dealing with it since then. Elizabeth kept telling herself she needed to slow down and that she was putting too much pressure on herself to perform and cross things off the list. She wanted to show the board how effective she was by completing her to-do list in months instead of years.

When Elizabeth met with her mentor, he couldn't believe what she was trying to do. He was a retired and successful superintendent for fifteen years in a neighboring school district. He said what she was attempting to do was unrealistic and was disingenuous to herself, as she was putting herself into a situation that wouldn't lead to anything positive. He tried to convince her to slow down, but she kept pushing forward. She wanted to prove something, but no one expected her to do what she was trying to do.

Now, Elizabeth wishes she had listened to her mentor. If she had, she wouldn't be in the situation she now finds herself in. She will more than likely, according to her physician, experience chronic migraines the rest of her life, because she continues to work at speeds that she knows are not sustainable. She completed her list of things in a little over a year, but at the cost of her health. She keeps telling herself that one day she will slow down, only to then tell herself she only has a few years to retire, so she speeds up and works even harder.

The board never put any pressure on Elizabeth to work like she was. She has a problem where she needs to work faster, harder, and longer than anyone else. Though she knows that she is hurting herself by doing so, she can't help but keep doing it. She tells herself that she will slow down tomorrow, but she never does. She has worked herself to a point where she stays in a regular state of stress, which triggers even more stress and more severe migraines.

Elizabeth can slow down at any time. She worries that she is in this perpetual cycle where she can't slow down until it's too late. She controls her work schedule but cannot bring herself to slow down, even when she experiences the most severe migraines. Her doctors keep pleading with her to slow down, as the medication is not going to solve her health issues if she continues to put her health in a constant pattern of stress. Her physicians often tell her, "Don't try to be a superwoman, just a superintendent," which is all the job requires.

Key Takeaway

Superhuman strength may lead to being a hero, but that does not mean you are a leader. Though superintendents, like principals and teachers, are heroes to many, no one expects them to be superhuman. Superintendents are human and therefore will experience failure, disappointment, and obstacles, which make them better and more realistic leaders. The most effective leaders don't try to be superhuman, they only lead and know their limitations.

Leaders commit to a life of service to others. One of the most important things a superintendent can do to serve others is to model the way for others of how not to be superhuman. Superintendents who try to be superman put pressure on others to also be superhuman with their actions. This isn't healthy for the superintendents, principals, teachers, or staff members in the district. There is nothing wrong with students, parents, or communities believing superintendents are heroes. The problem only develops when superintendents believe they must possess superhuman abilities and powers to serve their communities.

Something to think about is that when superintendents believe they are superhuman, they are destined for failure. There are no guarantees in life, but a superintendent who believes that they can be everywhere and everything to everybody is destined to fail. Unrealistic goals always start out meaning well but usually leave a leader questioning why, after failing, and wishing that they would have done things differently, often too late.

Students, teachers, staff members, parents, and members of the community need leadership, not necessarily heroism. You are human and, like your students, teachers, staff, parents, and community members, do not have unlimited sources of strength. You need time to replenish your body, because if you're not careful you can burn out quickly. Though you are looked to for leadership, you hurt and experience all the things that everyone does. There is no need to put on the facade you are superman or superwoman. The job only requires that you give your best each day—nothing more, nothing less.

CHAPTER EIGHTEEN

The Missed Art of Happiness

"The art of being happy lies in the power of extracting happiness from common things."

—Henry Ward Beecher

The chief executive officers of school districts, superintendents, have a lot on their shoulders each day. Decisions, answering questions, planning, meetings, counseling, communicating, and interacting with members of the community. The list could go on. What is missing from the list is focusing on the understanding of being happy. Too many superintendents each day find themselves staring into an abyss, a sea of darkness, with little hope of finding the light at the end of the tunnel. This is caused by leaders misunderstanding happiness. Happiness is not the lack of hardship but the mastery of it.

The position of superintendent is demanding, and, if not kept in perspective, can have crippling side effects on a superintendent's emotional, mental, and physical health, which impacts their well-being. Leaders need to be hopeful given the many stresses on their attitude and personality that come with being the superintendent. No one will find a school district with a healthy culture and an unhappy superintendent. It is that simple. The leader's emotional and mental health can and will have a tremendous impact on the school district, specifically, on student achievement, staff engagement, community support, and board effectiveness.

Employees want and need a leader who is positive, because it provides a sense of hope, which is one of the four basic needs of followers. Employees who have a positive and happy leader far outperform those employees with leaders who are negative and unhappy. Why? Happiness and unhappiness are contagious. When a leader is happy, they rub off on their employees as they work to create a culture that is inviting, inclusive, positive, and driven by a sense of hope.

Happiness is not solely focused on performance. Happiness isn't included in the health and well-being conversation solely to improve the performance of the school district. Happiness is mentioned because it has a direct effect on the superintendent's overall health and well-being. People who are naturally happier live longer, age more slowly, have fewer illnesses, are more active, and feel more confident about today and tomorrow. Furthermore, and this is big, happiness also reduces stress and anxiety, which both come with the job.

When happiness is mentioned, this doesn't mean that the superintendent must come into work jolly, outgoing, and with a pep in their step every day. They realize happiness is not about being all cheery and bright, but rather it is the simple harmony between a person and the life they live. This is why happiness comes in many shades and is tailored to each leader. Happiness will be exhibited differently from one superintendent to the next, but the important thing to keep in mind is that happiness shows up as hope. As superintendent are you happy personally and professionally? Do you enjoy going to work or are you stressed, angry, and depressed? Do you get personal enjoyment from the job?

One thing about happiness is no one can fake it. A person is either happy or they're not. Employees instinctively sense when their leader is happy, angry, stressed, depressed, and distant. It is important that the superintendent has a self-checkup each day before arriving to the office. Superintendents must be emotionally, mentally, socially, and physically prepared to lead. To be clear, no one can lead effectively without a certain level of happiness. Though this may seem too much like a "kumbaya" moment, happiness is real and critically important to the superintendent's health, as well as the health of the organization.

At the end of the day, superintendents must make their happiness a key staple of their leadership. Before they can lead effectively, they must make sure their talents match the demands of the role they are in. To deliver on the followers' need for hope, superintendents need to make sure that they get themselves healthy and whole. Additionally, they need to really make sure that they enjoy the job . . . the superintendency. If they are not happy—it happens—they need to make a personal decision to find a job that makes them happy. Staying in a job that makes one unhappy can have long-term negative impacts on one's health and well-being. It is not fair to the superintendent, their family, or their school district.

Practical Strategies

1. *Make time to reflect or perform a self-checkup in the morning.* As soon as you wake up each morning check yourself emotionally and mentally. Think about what state of mind you are in. Are you looking forward to the job each day or not? Are you tired, stressed, or depressed? Taking the time to perform a self-checkup can help you emotionally and mentally prepare for the day. You may need time to get yourself ready for the day. But know where you are emotionally, mentally, and physically each day before arriving to work.
2. *Focus on the things of the job that make you happy.* A lot of times superintendents focus on all the dreadful things that lead to elevated stress, anxiety, depression, and even burnout. But there are important things, such as speaking with students, helping teachers, having lunch with students, and interacting with employees and the community, that can bring you happiness to your job. If you feel you are dealing with more things that are stressful, sprinkle in things that make you happy as often as you can.
3. *Always wear your happiness.* Though a leader who wears their happiness positively impacts their employees, the purpose is not solely about the employee. If superintendents start their day off smiling, walking into the office greeting people, and laughing, the results show they are more likely to say their day was productive and fulfilling. Laughter has a self-healing power, and superintendents who say they laugh regularly throughout the day indicate they feel less stressed and find the job more rewarding.

Voices from the Field

The Cost of Unhappiness

Dr. Miguel Pertina is a sixty-three-year-old male, with close to twenty years of experience as a superintendent of a large school district in the Southwest. As most superintendents are still male, talking about happiness is a little out of character. As a male, Miguel was taught from an early age, like most men of his generation, that men work and never complain about their mental or physical health.

In fact, Miguel can't remember one time when his father said he was too sick, depressed, or not mentally right to go to work. Superintendents, likewise, are trained to focus on everyone else's well-being, and if they have time, they can then focus on their well-being. Like many, Miguel struggled with finding a balance between work and family and, more importantly, making sure he was emotionally, mentally, and physically okay to lead each day.

Talking about his health is always difficult for Miguel, even though he has come full circle with talking about his happiness. He has been a superintendent for twenty years in multiple districts. The current district where Miguel is superintendent will be his last stop, as he plans to retire in a couple of years if the board votes to renew his contract one last time. He would like to believe that his twenty years as a superintendent have been filled every day with happiness, but that has not been the case. He takes pride in serving as superintendent, but it has not come without a toll on his health and family.

Several years ago, Dr. Pertina went through a rough patch. When he reflects on those years, it seemed as if he woke up every day dreading the day. On some days he was just so emotionally and mentally drained that he didn't leave the house. The people at the district office were fantastic, and the board was very understanding of Miguel's situation as the job was draining him emotionally, mentally, and physically.

Furthermore, Miguel's mother and father passed away within a few months of each other, which had a significant impact on him. He would visit with them as often as he could and enjoyed spending time sitting around their dining room table with his parents, brothers, and sisters. Also, Miguel was going through a divorce, and he takes full responsibility for that as well. He was working so much; his wife would only see him for a couple of minutes in the evening and a few hours over the weekend.

Dr. Pertina's schedule became so consumed by the job that he began to get home in the evenings and not realize on many occasions that his wife had bought new furniture for the living room. He simply did not see it. He was so consumed by the job he didn't realize what was going on around him at work or at home. Eventually, his wife asked for a divorce because she became tired of never seeing him and trying to live with only a few minutes or hours per week. Many superintendents' marriages end in divorce because of the job, but it doesn't have to be this way.

During the year, Miguel was so unhappy. He can't remember if he smiled or laughed a single day. If he did, it was extraordinarily rare. He felt his job, as superintendent, was to go to work every day, work long hours, take care of others, and never complain about what he was going through personally or professionally. The job, in combination with the loss of his parents and his divorce, became too much to handle. He wasn't leading, and he was barely surviving at that point.

It took Miguel some time to realize that he needed to focus on himself so he could be there for others. At first, he started out angry for allowing himself to get to this state. After anger, he then moved to feeling sorry for himself. He eventually came to terms with the fact that he wasn't okay, and he needed to figure out why. Still to this day, he contends that if he had only slowed down earlier and recognized he wasn't going to work because he enjoyed the job but more out of compliance and trying to live up to the same working terms his father did, he would not have become depressed and he would not have lost his wife.

Dr. Pertina had to come to terms with the fact that he wasn't happy. Furthermore, he wasn't healthy emotionally or mentally. He wanted to be happy, but he had to overcome deeply ingrained beliefs about what was expected of him. Furthermore, he had to have some closure with his parents passing away, as the job didn't allow him time to grieve appropriately.

Miguel didn't have to work each day to exhaustion. He could take vacations, and on some days, he needed some time just for himself to rejuvenate his emotional and mental health. He realized that it didn't take a degree in rocket science to figure out happiness. All he needed to do was to slow down, enjoy each day, focus on what he enjoyed the most as superintendent, and realize the opportunities that existed in life. In the past, he lived to work. Now, he works to live.

Key Takeaway

Happiness can exist in the life of a superintendent. The key is simple but elusive to many school leaders, especially right now based on all the things they must navigate (e.g., COVID-19) as a leader. To experience happiness, superintendents must slow down and enjoy life and the job. Superintendents can't go at breakneck speed every day and expect to experience happiness. Furthermore, this pace of going from one meeting to the next, working eighty-plus hours per week, never taking vacations only charts a path with a disastrous and tragic outcome.

No superintendent should have to go to work each day with feelings of unhappiness. The job is one of the best jobs, but the key is to control your own schedule as much as possible. Additionally, superintendents must recognize the importance of focusing on their own emotional, mental, and physical well-being. If there is a misalignment between the job and the superintendent's health, including their happiness, superintendents can't be successful or effective, and will eventually burn out and leave the profession.

Too many superintendents arrive at work and go through life in search of fulfillment and happiness but never find it because they become trapped by the demands of the job. They continue to push forward, sometimes causing irreparable harm to themselves, because they believe the job demands their undivided attention all the time. This is no way to live or to lead and will never end with the superintendent finding happiness. Yes, sometimes superintendents need to slow down and appreciate life and recalibrate their personal and professional lives so that they can experience happiness. That's leadership and life!

CHAPTER NINETEEN
Never Lose Hope or Abandon Your Dreams

"Don't be pushed by your problems. Be led by your dreams."
—Ralph Waldo Emerson

Many readers will undoubtedly find this chapter interesting and peculiar, as hopes and dreams are seldom discussed in terms of superintendent self-care. Both are something to discuss in terms of self-care, but they are also integral to understanding each person's drive, goals, and opportunities to succeed. As the superintendency continues to grow in its complexities, hope and dreams make take a back seat to the demands of the job. You may have heard that a person who has lost hope or given up on their dreams is likely to give up on life.

The push and pull of the job, the role of superintendent, is hard on every man and woman who currently holds or has had held the position. No matter the size or location of your school district, from time to time there will be moments when you want to give up. The job begins to drown you, making you believe there is no hope, and your dreams become distant wishes. Physically you may be doing okay, but mentally and emotionally you are slowly killing yourself. A person without hope or dreams is destined for severe health complications.

Superintendents are so focused on everyone else and their surroundings that they forget about hope and their dreams. Likewise, many forget to carve out some time during the day to focus on their health and well-being. Hope and dreams are tickets to a renewed feeling of satisfaction, success, and peace of mind. Both are antidepressants to many, including superintendents.

There are so many examples of leaders losing hope, forgetting their dreams, and experiencing severe panic attacks or mental breakdowns leading to hospitalizations. Just like our bodies, our minds can only take so much. Eventually, the body will begin to shut down as a safety mechanism to prevent long-term damage. Heed this warning: Once you lose hope and forget about your dreams, recovery is long and, in some cases, not possible at all.

Have you ever sat behind your desk in your office and tried to think about tomorrow or review your dreams? Though every superintendent's schedule is tight each day, with only a few minutes, if any, allocated for themselves, it's critical to find a healthy work-life balance. There is nothing wrong with closing your door, putting down your cell phone, pushing paperwork to the side, and turning off the monitor to your desktop for several minutes throughout the day to give your mind and body a break.

These breaks throughout the day are rejuvenating for your mind, body, spirit, and soul. Stress is kryptonite to hope and dreams, and it's bountiful in the superintendency. The superintendency is a minefield of stress that is peaking around every corner, and the sooner superintendents recognize this detriment the better. Stress is a major force that is still being researched in the medical field in an attempt to discover just how impactful it can be on a person's health.

It is fitting that this chapter started with a simple quote by Ralph Waldo Emerson. Though the quote is simple and concise, it is so true and speaks volumes to every superintendent. Every day, superintendents, servant leaders by nature of the office, try to extinguish multiple fires, chart varying paths for the future, and interact with countless numbers of people. In other words, they solve problems. These problems—few small, most large—always end up on the desk of the superintendent, hence the inevitability of too many superintendents being driven by problems and less by their dreams.

Superintendents must change the dynamics of the job if they expect to survive the daunting and sometimes overwhelming responsibilities that accompany the office. Not only will superintendents become better leaders if they exhibit hope and dream more but their overall health and well-being will also be drastically changed . . . for the better. Quite frankly, a person cannot be a leader if they lack hope and fail to dream. Furthermore, life seems a little drearier if there is no hope of tomorrow or our dreams seem to fade.

Our minds, bodies, spirit, and soul are remarkable things. All are prerequisites to a healthy work-life balance. No matter how hopeless it may seem, all four are repairable for superintendents if they just take the time to rekindle the energies that brought them to this amazing office. Too often, superintendents are so programmed to focus on current or past problems, they forget about their hope and dreams of a better tomorrow for themselves and their school districts.

It is highly likely that few will agree that hope and dreams have anything to do with health and well-being. Those who don't are more than likely already struggling with and will suffer from an eventual crippling work-life balance. Can you imagine a person, a leader, who lacks hope and dreams? Hope and dreams matter just as much as the other Xs and Os that we would normally equate to health and well-being, such as diet, exercise, sleep, water, and spirituality. Never underestimate the transformative power of hope and dreams to your personal and professional life. More importantly, keep hoping and dreaming—for your sake and the sake of the students, teachers, and staff that you lead each day.

Practical Strategies

1. *Write down your hope and dreams.* No matter whether you are a novice or veteran superintendent, start the job or start a new day by writing down your hope and dreams. Once you have them written down, make sure to place them in a prominent spot in your office to remind you each day. Some superintendents even carry them in their wallets, purses, or briefcases and bags. When your world seems a little less bright, look at the piece of paper or card and make sure you stay grounded by your hopes and dreams.

2. *Make your health part of your hopes and dreams.* Don't think it's too late to change. Be hopeful that you can make changes in your life, diet, exercise routine, and professional commitments. Your journey to a healthy well-being starts with goals or dreams no matter who you are. Take each step of the journey one by one but be aware of setbacks that may derail you or encourage you to quit. Your hopes and dreams are powerful motivating factors to your overall health.

3. *Ensure your hopes and dreams are meaningful and realistic.* They should encourage you to keep pushing forward. No matter how debilitating your health is, always have hope for a better tomorrow. Hopes and dreams aren't about winning the lottery and retiring from the profession—that is too superficial. Meaningful hopes and dreams are important to you, your family, and your career.

Voices from the Field

Hope Isn't a Given

Rosalyn Fromm is a sixty-year-old, eighteen-year veteran superintendent of a large and diversified school district in the Midwest. Hope of a better tomorrow doesn't always come easy for a superintendent, especially over the past two years having to navigate so many uncertainties in education and the community. Truth be told, hope is a topic that isn't paid much attention to in preparation programs to become a superintendent.

Rosalyn can't remember one time when hope was mentioned in a course or part of an assignment when she was completing her graduate degree to become a superintendent. Likewise, a quick review of superintendent preparation programs proves that health and well-being are not mentioned or minimally referenced. As part of health and well-being, hope is critical to the success of a superintendent.

Rosalyn remembers that over the course of her extensive career as a school principal and superintendent, the job would get out of control and thus would allow her health to get out of control. Though her health is the best it has been in several years, she struggles with her diet, exercise, and finding the proper balance between life and work. Each time her health gets out of control, her hopes and dreams also seem distant or not as clear.

Mrs. Fromm often feels depressed and fatigued. She often tells new or aspiring superintendents that when it comes to hope and dreams, they must be part of their daily focus. There are so many more things to life than the superintendency. If there aren't clear parameters set for work, life, and health, it is easy for superintendents to become absorbed by the job before they realize what is happening.

The job allows Rosalyn to get so entrenched in the day-to-day processes of the superintendency, that her health starts to slide if she is not careful. When her schedule is booked solid, she feels the onset of anxiety, body aches, headaches, fatigue, and some depression. When this happens, the thought or hope of a better tomorrow seems disingenuous, as she is just trying to survive the day. By the time she arrives home in the evening from the office, she just wants to be left alone and prefers silence. She is emotionally, mentally, and physically drained, and all she keeps thinking about is her schedule tomorrow.

The job of the superintendent is emotionally, mentally, and physically draining for every superintendent. After a couple of days of depression, Rosalyn is able to balance her schedule. Her balanced schedule allows her to be a leader, mom, wife, and friend. She considers herself a positive person who tries to convey a sense of hope and encourages others to follow their dreams.

The pressures of the job at times are overwhelming, yet people need her to be able to steer the ship in the right direction. She knows that to help others have hope and follow their dreams, her health must be made a priority. It is so easy for health and well-being to be placed on the backburner, but each time that happens, the parade of horrible begins.

Some superintendents are aware of the importance of maintaining a positive work-life balance and can quickly control what is happening. Unfortunately, those who are not aware experience a variety of health issues, as well as problems at home due to an unhealthy work-life balance. No superintendent is perfect, and everyone from time to time will allow their health to drop down on their priority list.

Though Rosalyn experiences periods of declining focus on her health, she now recognizes her pressure points and understands the importance of health to her overall success. No superintendent can lead effectively if their health is out of control. Sadly, too many superintendents go their entire careers without ever recognizing how important their health is or they get on the proverbial hamster wheel, working nonstop each day with little focus on what they eat or how much sleep they get. They think they are being successful, which may be true, but eventually, their health catches up to them and their hope fades.

Key Takeaway

Never underestimate the power of having hope and dreams in terms of your success as a leader and maintaining your health. The health of a leader is paramount to the health of the organization. When leaders are healthy the organization is healthy and vice versa. All of this begins with the leader's hope and dreams. The healthiest leaders recognize the importance of maintaining their hopes and dreams as relevant in their daily schedule.

Instead of being jam-packed with meetings from start to finish with little or no time for themselves, leaders should have the expectation that they have time for themselves throughout the day. This time is for reflection, exercise, or disconnecting from the job or life. Exercise, time alone, and turning off phones allow leaders to maintain a focus on their health and their hopes and dreams. Health and well-being aren't always determined by diet, exercise, and sleep. Hope and dreams, though they are hard to visualize and touch, need to be exercised routinely to maintain a healthy well-being.

CHAPTER TWENTY

Exercise and Leadership: The Missing Connection

"Those who think they have no time for exercise will sooner or later have to find time for illness."

—Edward Stanley

Superintendents often believe that they do not have the luxury to make time for their health and well-being. Many are rushing from one meeting to the next and one crisis to the next, all the while forgetting about just how important their health and well-being are to their success and the long-term success of the district they are charged to lead. Superintendents often overlook this crucial element of being an effective leader: their own health and well-being.

There is so much more to leadership than the normal Xs and Os from the training manual that most superintendents read from. For far too long, superintendents have been squarely focused on their well-doing (performance) with little focus on their well-being. For decades, since the start of high-stakes testing and especially after the passage of No Child Left Behind (NCLB), most superintendents have been focused on test scores (well-doing).

Everything throughout a superintendent's day has been rearranged to prioritize test scores. As this started consuming the superintendent's day and focus, the health and well-being of students, teachers, and staff, including their own, were moved to the backburner and forgotten. The addiction of "doing" overwhelmed the need for our well-being. Schools and society are now reaping the outcomes of high-stakes testing, which is why stress among students, teachers, and leaders has skyrocketed over the past decades.

Exercise is a release and an investment for some superintendents. They realize physical well-being is about managing their health so that they have the energy to do all the things they want to do. Those few superintendents who have prioritized their health and well-being continue to speak about how transformative it has been for them personally and as a leader. Instead of focusing solely on well-doing, these few superintendents have prioritized well-being, and it resonates in the culture of the school district.

In those school districts, well-being is a prerequisite for better outcomes and improved performance. Those superintendents understand that they are more effective as leaders when their bodies, minds, and souls are healthy. They also understand, as the leader, that this is a key component of their effort to "Model the Way." People want and expect leaders to model the way in so many aspects of life, including health, well-being, and exercise.

On the totem pole of priorities, exercise, health, and well-being are often missing for superintendents for several reasons. First, it is not simply the lack of wanting to exercise; they just don't know where and how to start. They haven't exercised in years, so they start exercising without a well-developed plan and suddenly stop due to a lack of know-how. Second, superintendents set unrealistic goals, thinking they can transform themselves overnight.

This isn't just with superintendents, but most who start exercising believe they can see overnight successes. When the overnight results don't happen, they stop and give up. Being physically active should not merely be a goal. It must become a way of life. The good news is that, per recent research, even a small amount of physical activity (of any kind) boosts happiness almost immediately. Even those who exercise two days a week are happier and have significantly less stress. More effective than prescription drugs, exercising is also one of the best ways to combat fatigue. In fact, exercise improves mood, immunity, and learning.

Third, like most adults, many superintendents buy into the idea that exercising has to be "fancy" or "as seen on TV," joining commercial gyms, purchasing exercise programs, or buying extravagant equipment. Again, in most cases, superintendents stop going to their monthly membership gyms, stop watching their exercise programs, and allow dust to collect on their new expensive equipment after only a few uses.

The last reason superintendents do not exercise is they feel as if they do not have the time to do so. Most superintendents make time for everything pertaining to the job, but rarely for important things such as exercise, health, and their families. They fall victim to the notion that exercise or time alone with friends or family weakens their ability to lead. But in fact, it is the exact opposite.

Superintendents who have found a schedule that includes exercise are more present in life, healthier, and far more effective in their roles than those who continue to struggle to find a healthy work-life balance. Superintendents often focus on the traditional things of leadership and fail to consider just how important the softer things, such as health and well-being impact their overall effectiveness.

Keep in mind that exercise doesn't have to be fancy or sophisticated to be effective. Finding time to walk, jog, run, swim, lift weights, or golf (not riding in the cart) can be done easily and cheaply. Likewise, exercise doesn't have to be complicated. There are abundant free exercise plans that can be done in the comfort of your home on the Internet. Exercise doesn't require much to be effective. For instance, jumping rope three to four times a week, costs a few dollars but can have positive life effects.

Leadership and exercise share an inherent bond. Like leadership, to be effective, exercise must be made a priority and performed consistently. Neither leadership nor exercise happens by chance. Both take commitment, strategy, and understanding. Without commitment, exercise will be a one-and-done event. Likewise, without a strategy, exercise will not result in desired outcomes and could end with a life-altering injury.

Finally, without understanding just how important exercise is to one's well-being, a leader will soon regret missed opportunities and wish things were different when it may be too late. A superintendent must not discount how important exercise, along with establishing a healthy work-life balance, is to their overall effectiveness as a leader. The superintendency has a way of pulling a person into a cycle that is not healthy.

Though there are numerous superintendents who have been in the position for years without prioritizing their health and well-being, including never or seldomly exercising, they are few and far between. Superintendents today face more stress, work longer hours, and face unthinkable situations, such as a global health pandemic. Without a release like exercising, their tenures as superintendents will be short-lived. It's inevitable.

Prioritizing exercise improves mood, immunity, and learning. Superintendents must never believe it takes away from their ability to lead effectively. When leadership and exercise are practiced in unison, there isn't a give and take, but a successful equation for longevity and effectiveness and a positive work-life balance. Though finding the balance is difficult at times and many will never find this balance, it exists and is much needed by superintendents for the benefit of themselves and those they are leading.

Exercise, like leadership, is a journey. There are no overnight transformations. Both require superintendents to make time for their development. As leadership is about growth, exercise provides the ability, energy, and path for growth to occur. Superintendents want to lead for years, but without their health, which requires a certain level of exercise, their hopes and wishes for longevity rarely come to fruition. Though many superintendents say they do not have time to focus on their health, the question becomes how they could not, if health and well-being are mission-critical to their success as a superintendent.

Practical Strategies

1. *Start slow.* The first rule of thumb is to start slow. Superintendents shouldn't start by trying to run a marathon if they have not ever run one before or haven't run in years. Start with small goals. For instance, if the ultimate goal is to run a marathon, start off running, slowly, for ten to fifteen minutes, working your way up in incremental steps. Starting slow and increasing the length of the run over time, instead of overnight, will help the body to become acclimated, including by building muscle strength and lung capacity.

2. *Be realistic.* Commercialized exercise programs, though they may have good intentions, will often lead to unrealistic expectations and goals. There are few, if any, programs that can result in magazine-cover abdominal muscles or biceps. The goal of exercising is to improve your health, not necessarily to obtain the physique of Mr. or Mrs. Universe. Furthermore, when starting out, the smaller the goals the better. Quick, small wins create the foundation for longer, bigger wins.

3. *Do it, but don't overdo it.* Think about how many people start exercising on January 1 every year and give up by the end of the week. Again, it's about starting slow and small. Depending on many factors, using a five-pound dumbbell and starting out with more repetitions is more effective than a heavier and uncontrollable weight with fewer repetitions. Overdoing it after years of not exercising can result in giving up quickly and severe injuries, both of which are counterproductive to the goal of exercise.

4. *Schedule time.* There are many variations to exercise. Some will prefer to exercise before going to the office, while others prefer after work. There may even be a few who have the luxury of exercising throughout the workday. No matter the preference, make exercise a regular

appointment on the calendar and be very protective of this time. No one can change without approval! Again, schedule things that matter!

5. *Communicate importance.* Superintendents must start by communicating the importance of their health and well-being to members of the board. Explain to the board how important exercise is to you to become an effective leader in the district. Most boards will understand and support prioritizing your health and well-being, as most boards want stability in the position, and that requires longevity, which requires health.

Voices from the Field

Exercising Leadership

Dr. Demetrius Cooper is a forty-three-year-old who has been a superintendent for the past four years of an urban school district in the upper Midwest. He has always enjoyed exercising. He played basketball from elementary school through college and continues to do so even as a superintendent, joining local pick-up games around town with friends. When he can't play basketball, Demetrius is seen in the high school weight room.

When the local board of education hired Dr. Cooper, he was clear on how important his health was to him as a father and husband. He explained that his father passed away due to a heart attack when he was only forty-eight years old, and he is trying to make sure that his health is always at the forefront so he can live to see his son and daughter grow up. By communicating to the board from the beginning just how important his health was to him, the board was fully aware of his expectations.

Often superintendents believe that the work comes before everything else, but with Dr. Cooper, his health and family come before work, as it should be. Though it is difficult to arrange priorities due to the demands and pressures of the job, superintendents must be upfront with the board of education about their priorities and work each day to prioritize their schedule to accommodate their health.

Each day, Demetrius wakes up early, goes down his basement, and either lifts weights or runs on the treadmill. He arrives at work refreshed and ready to start the day. He tells colleagues that on days he isn't able to work out or run, his day seems odd. He admits that on some days his schedule gets out of control, but he quickly works to make it manageable. On days that he isn't able to work out or run, he tries to go to the local basketball court and joins in a pick-up game. He is also a regular at the men's basketball practice, joining in with student-athletes practicing, which the head coach says is an awesome experience for students.

Demetrius is one of those leaders who tries to model the way for others. Yes, his health is important to him, but he is also concerned about the health and well-being of students, teachers, and staff in the district. When he visits schools, he always visits the physical education classes to see what students are learning about exercise. He is known for giving a few pointers to students and teachers during these informal walkthroughs.

Likewise, Dr. Cooper talks to teachers and staff about their health and well-being. He encourages walking professional learning communities (PLC) meetings, as too many meetings lead to too much sitting around, which isn't good for teachers' or administrators' health, and walking encourages creativity and innovation. Furthermore, at least once a month, Dr. Cooper purchases fruit, healthy snacks, and bottles of water for staff and places the items in the workroom or breakroom. He doesn't just talk about the importance of health; he models the importance of health to stakeholders in his district.

Many superintendents believe that when they take their eyes off the ball—the office—they begin to lose control or effectiveness. Dr. Cooper is different. He believes that his leadership is more effective because he has prioritized his health, and the board of education agrees. Each of his annual evaluations has been rated as exemplary, and in fact, the board applauds publicly and privately how well he manages his time, includes stakeholders in decision-making, and has prioritized the health and well-being of stakeholders.

Key Takeaway

There will always be some excuse that can keep a superintendent from focusing on their health and well-being. The demands and stresses of the superintendency will only increase over the coming years, so if leaders do not find a way now to exercise and focus on their health and well-being, then they are less likely to do so tomorrow. Superintendents must stop thinking a focus on their health takes away from their ability to lead.

In fact, it is the exact opposite. Prioritizing health and well-being, including exercise, will only strengthen your leadership abilities. Superintendents are faced with countless decisions each day. The decision to exercise, to prioritize their health and well-being, is not one of those decisions. The problem and difficulty, for many superintendents, stems from a lack of understanding of how and when to start.

Exercise is difficult for the majority of adults and leaders; it is not a phenomenon just within the superintendency. The key is to start small and slow after establishing realistic goals and with an understanding that it is a marathon and not a race, as results never occur overnight. You can't rush progress or change. Though change may take time, especially with repairing your health and well-being, don't become discouraged. Keep pushing forward.

Superintendents must realize that exercise isn't about developing magazine-cover physiques, but rather it is about establishing, improving, and strengthening their healthy work-life balance. Exercise combined with a healthy diet and sleep schedule can do wonders for any superintendent. The one thing to remember is that exercise, for thirty to forty-five minutes a day before or after work, can have many positive outcomes for each superintendent. The only requirement is to take the first step and begin exercising. Running, going for a walk after work, playing golf, lifting weights, riding a bicycle, or swimming is all that is needed, and in many cases, it costs nothing and only demands a few minutes a week to be transformative personally and professionally.

CHAPTER TWENTY-ONE

Prevention, Not a Reaction

"True prevention is not waiting for bad things to happen; it's preventing things from happening in the first place."

—Don McPherson

Superintendents, like most adults, are terrible at recognizing their health, especially when their health is on the decline. Most adults will only make health a priority after an accident or health scare. The American healthcare system is designed to address problems after the fact, not necessarily before. Adults are comfortable with putting their health on the backburner while pushing forward with their jobs.

This mindset has only led to an increase in severe health conditions among adults, including superintendents. The best way to remain a superintendent is to make sure that health is a priority before the job begins to not damage overall health and well-being. The superintendency requires long hours, brings a lot of stress and anxiety, and allows for extraordinarily little personal time.

With so many things happening each day, most superintendents struggle with finding time for themselves, including preventative healthcare. A simple checkup with a physician seems next to impossible some days, but the importance of such meetings cannot be overstated. If you look at Fortune 500 companies, the top executives make their health a priority. Though it may be difficult to compare the job of a superintendent with a Fortune 500 executive, there are similarities.

For this discussion, the similarities are similar in terms of leading employees, budgetary considerations, work schedules, and health. Both the business executive and superintendent are responsible not only for the health of the organization, including employees, but also for their own health. Unfortunately, most superintendents have failed to recognize just how important their overall health and well-being are to their employee's well-being and the health of the organization.

Superintendents have a job that brings massive responsibilities, and, at the end of the day, they are responsible for the country's most precious asset—students, tomorrow's future. Often, superintendents feel as if the weight of the world is on their shoulders. But that doesn't mean that throughout the pressures, they cannot focus on their own well-being. It is quite simple; unhealthy well-being directly impacts the overall effectiveness of any leader. Superintendents who allow the job to control their life and, in doing so, allow their health to take a backseat, are destined to fail.

Prevention seems like a foreign term to superintendents. They are good at reacting to a situation but find it exceedingly difficult to practice prevention. There are so many things that superintendents confront on any given day, but their health is often not one of them. If prevention is a foreign term to superintendents, then preventative healthcare is a completely different universe of thinking.

Prevention takes time, and superintendents struggle with an already packed daily schedule. But the more they schedule preventative health checkups, time for exercise, relaxation, family, and a healthy diet, the more time they have in the end. This will be difficult for many to believe or grasp, but prevention is cheaper, allows for more time, improves focus, and enhances effectiveness and performance.

Superintendents must slow down and prioritize preventative healthcare. The more they get ahead of their health, the better they will be able to lead. It's amazing how many superintendents will allow themselves to reach the point of exhaustion and then ask why they don't feel well or feel unhealthy. Exhaustion should not be the only time a superintendent thinks about their health. But to be clear, the more often a superintendent reaches a point of exhaustion or is crippled by some health condition, the closer they become to a point of no return.

Reactionary healthcare is a Band-Aid to a larger issue that will only work for so long. If a superintendent, once they are feeling better, returns to the job and resumes the same work style with no changes, more damage is done to their health, and the possibility of a more severe health outcome increases. Superintendents will not be one for long if they continue to burn both ends of the candle. The saying "an ounce of prevention is worth a pound of cure," is precisely the mindset that must be developed among superintendents.

Superintendents cannot continue to operate as they had in the past, as if they are immortal. Eventually, their health will get to the point where they are forced to address their health and well-being. Unfortunately, for many, by the time they do make their health a focus, it's too late. Preventative healthcare is something new to many but must become the standard practice for superintendents. This goes well beyond regular checkups and must include a focus on the superintendent's emotional, mental, and physical well-being.

Practical Strategies

1. *Find a physician that focuses on preventative healthcare.* A preventative physician specializes in stress, fatigue, diet, and overall health associated with the workplace. They understand the pressures of the job and can help design a preventative regimen that aligns with the job but also takes care of your health. Don't be afraid to seek help if the job becomes overwhelming and you recognize your health and well-being are being jeopardized.
2. *Know your limits and change paths when the job becomes too much.* If you are working too much, recognize what it is doing to your health, family, and friends. When you reach a brick wall with your health, it is not advisable to push through. Seek help. But more importantly, never reach the brick wall. No one expects superintendents to work to the point of exhaustion, which leads to permanent health issues.
3. *Schedule "you time" throughout the school day.* This is your time to disconnect from technology—yes, your cell phone included—and focus on you for at least fifteen to twenty minutes each day. These few minutes are like a wonder drug to your overall health. If you can squeeze in time for yourself during the morning and afternoon, the effects will be remarkable in terms of your performance and overall health and well-being.

Voices from the Field

An Ounce of Prevention Is Worth a Pound of Cure

Dr. Tabitha Whitaker is a fifty-two-year-old who has been the superintendent of a rural school district located in the Southeast for the past seven years. Superintendents in just a few years are exposed to so many leadership experiences. Though Dr. Whitaker is in her fifth year as a superintendent, she is considered a veteran superintendent in her state. This is becoming normal across the nation as more superintendents leave the profession. However, she does not consider herself an expert or a veteran.

Dr. Whitaker is a good example of a superintendent who didn't realize how much stress she was placing on herself. Like many superintendents, she thought she could handle any of the stresses that the job presented and was willing to work through them. Now she understands superintendents who are struggling with their job and their health, as she also went through the same experience.

Tabitha is the first to acknowledge that she is not perfect, and at one point in time, she allowed her health to get to a point where she experienced a mild heart attack at the age of forty-nine. It took a scare, like a heart attack, to get her attention and help her to realize that burning both ends of the candlestick never pays off. Unfortunately, too many superintendents don't realize that prevention is key to longevity.

At the time of Dr. Whitaker's heart attack, she was working like she was immortal. She rarely took time off for anything, and if she was sick, she still showed up to work. The only time she took off was to attend the funeral of her grandfather who lived in another state. Otherwise, she was working five to seven days a week for at least three years, until her body couldn't take it anymore. It wasn't just her physical health; her emotional health was suffering just as much as her physical health.

Tabitha spent a week in the hospital as the doctors tried to get her heart back in rhythm. As she reflects, she was working so much, trying to be at work every day and ultimately jeopardized her health. She had placed unrealistic goals on herself, and the return was a damaged heart at forty-nine years old. Today, she can't believe she put her body through this amount of stress, but she now recognizes the importance of preventative health strategies.

While in the hospital, Dr. Whitaker's cardiologist suggested that she contact a specialist that deals with preventative healthcare for professionals. Even as a cardiologist, like him, he tended to allow his health to get out of control. He now goes to the specialist regularly to help hold him accountable for his own health. He referred Tabitha to the specialist and had her first appointment scheduled for the next week after she was discharged from the hospital.

Dr. Whitaker attended her first meeting with Dr. Weber, and from then on, she changed her way of thinking as a superintendent. Dr. Weber is an internist but also a certified health coach and trainer. His practice focuses primarily on working professionals, helping them with preventative healthcare, such as diets, exercise, and counseling. Prior to attending her first appointment, she thought this was going to be a one-time appointment at a fly-by-night doctor's office in some rundown medical facility.

Needless to say, Tabitha was wrong. The doctor's office was in a new medical office complex, and the waiting room was packed with professionals just like her, and it was at 1:00 p.m. during the workday. Her first meeting was a consultation with Dr. Weber, to allow him to assess her conditions. Her cardiologist had already sent over her file from the hospital. What she really liked was that he was not judgmental but more interested in what she was doing now to not get back into the shape she was in just a few weeks ago.

Over the course of two years, Dr. Weber helped Dr. Whitaker accept that it was okay for her to focus on her health and well-being. His goal was to help her to focus on her health and well-being before something, like a heart attack, happened again. Her appointments are twice a month and more like counseling sessions, as she discusses her workload and what she is doing to allow her mind and body time to heal and recover from a hectic day at the office. He performs normal checkups like blood pressure, temperature, breathing, and anything else she tells him about, but most of the session is focused on her overall health, dieting, and workload.

Dr. Weber requires Tabitha to keep a schedule and to bring it with her to each appointment. He helps her prioritize her health and the job. Again, if she is working long hours, he always asks how often she is exercising, what her diet looks like, and when she takes a break by doing something that she wants to do. Though she always felt doctors cared more about prescribing medications, Dr. Weber's interest is about her and helping her to focus on herself for a change.

Having been a patient of Dr. Weber's for two years, she can say that she feels healthier and is happier. Tabitha exercises at least four days a week. Prior to her heart attack, she wasn't exercising any because she didn't make time for herself. Plus, Dr. Weber helped her get her diet under control, as she was living off snacks and fast food prior to her heart attack. She snow spends Sunday afternoons prepping healthy meals and snacks for the upcoming week. She does not go into the office on Saturdays and Sundays any longer.

Many superintendents struggle balancing their job and health. It is important that superintendents begin focusing on preventative healthcare instead of waiting until something happens with their health that may not be reversible. Balancing the job and health isn't easy, and many superintendents will struggle at first finding time for themselves. But if they don't, they will end up just like Dr. Whitaker, experiencing a severe health condition prematurely.

Key Takeaway

If you don't think that you have time to focus on your health and well-being, life has an interesting way of making you make time. Too many superintendents don't prioritize their health until it's too late. Too many superintendents are dealing with heart issues, stress, obesity, mental issues, and other physical ailments all because of the pressures of the superintendency. Today, superintendents only react to their health when something goes wrong.

Superintendents must develop an understanding that preventive health strategies save a lot of money and time in the long run. Though, understandably, making time for themselves will be a foreign term for too many superintendents, it is imperative for superintendents to realize just how important their health and well-being is to their effectiveness as a leader. By slowing down and making your health and well-being a priority now, you will reap huge dividends as a superintendent and for your school district. Preventative strategies must become the standard for superintendents so that they can be better and healthier leaders, today and tomorrow.

CHAPTER TWENTY-TWO
Life After the Superintendency

"Most people work hard and spend their health trying to achieve wealth.
Then they retire and spend their wealth trying to get back their health."
—Kevin Gianni

This chapter of the book is a culminating message for all superintendents. No matter how hard a person works over their career as a superintendent or how committed they are to the job, there is never an excuse to jeopardize one's own health. Most superintendents when they retire have spent, on average, at least twenty to twenty-five years in education. Most have been in education all their lives, many in multiple states and districts.

There are some superintendents who have retired in one state and are now working as a superintendent in another state to boost their retirement and the enjoyment they get from working and leading in education. The opportunity to serve as superintendent even after one retires is appealing. Many superintendents go on after retirement to work as consultants, interim superintendents, superintendents, and leaders in other sectors.

This is not to say those superintendents who decide to accept a superintendent position after retirement are just doing it for the money. The pressures of the job and the daily grind are not as stress-filled in comparison to the superintendent who is trying to get to the point where they can retire. Hopefully, superintendents are not working to retire, only to fail at retirement and return to working long hours. Hopefully, their retirement is full of travel, grandkids, and doing things they want to do for a change. But their health is key to their happiness and mobility!

The daily grind of the superintendency is life-changing to many and even tragic for some. It is always heartbreaking to learn of a superintendent who passes away with only a few years before they can retire. Heart attack, stroke, and cancer, regularly associated with the passing of superintendents, all have strong connections to the overall health and well-being of superintendents. In many cases, stress, poor diet, lack of sleep, low levels of exercise, long hours, and elevated levels of anxiety all can lead to a shortened lifespan.

Too many superintendents get to the end of their careers and realize their bodies are wrecked. In many cases, superintendents must retire before they want to due to a crippling health condition. Once they retire, they spend the rest of their lives trying to get their health back, which without question, is much more difficult to do than when they started their education careers. We reap what we sow, and the harvest isn't promising for many superintendents who exhaust their bodies and minds.

It simply doesn't make sense, especially in today's superintendency, when there is so much research out about self-care, to constantly exhaust our bodies and minds for the job. This does not mean that superintendents shouldn't commit to the job fully. Boards of education, students, teachers, staff, parents, and the community need superintendents who are fully committed and not only involved (just counting the days to retirement or their next job).

To be clear, commitment does not mean that superintendents destroy or severely injure themselves emotionally, mentally, or physically for the job. No superintendent wants to retire only to find themselves spending most of their time dealing with lingering health issues caused by the job. The superintendency is not for the faint of heart or for those with health issues. The job has exacerbated the health of the strongest men and women.

But it doesn't have to be this way. Yes, superintendents are working to improve academic and nonacademic outcomes for students, but that doesn't mean they must work to the point of exhaustion, burnout, or physical impairment. Superintendents can change their health trajectory so that they can enjoy their life after the superintendents. There is nothing more important to the superintendency than the health and well-being of the leader.

Understandably, health and well-being are buried by the gravity of the job. In simple terms, superintendents must make their health and well-being just as important as every other responsibility of the job. The superintendency will never span the life of the leader; however, their health has a lot to do with their life span. It is obvious that exhaustion, stress, anxiety, depression, obesity, and high blood pressure do not lead to a longer life, yet so many superintendents succumb to these serious long-term health conditions.

If superintendents take nothing else from this book, they must understand that working to the point of mental or physical injury is not part of the job description. More importantly, poor health during the superintendency will not lead to a happy or healthy post-superintendency. Superintendents always talk about what they want to do after they retire: golf, go on trips, continue working in some other capacity, start a small business, or spend time with family and friends.

Sadly, too many superintendents' dreams take a back seat to their poor health. Life after the superintendency doesn't have to be filled with ongoing doctor's appointments, confined to using a walker or wheelchair, or wishing that you were in better health. You are always in control of your journey, including your journey to a healthy work-life balance. If you want to have an enjoyable life after the superintendency, start today, don't wait until tomorrow.

Every day that you put off your health is one less day once you retire that you will get to enjoy. This is not meant to scare anyone but instead to bring attention to an important facet of the superintendency. If you change your lifestyle and superintendency today, by focusing on your health and well-being, your life after you leave office will be far more rewarding. Yes, it's that simple!

Practical Strategies

1. *Find a physician that focuses on preventative health.* Superintendents, like most adults, only go to the doctor when something is wrong. Instead, superintendents should be focused on preventative health, scheduling regular checkups with their physicians. The trick is to find current or future problems early and address those health problems, rather than allowing them to get to an irreparable point. Medical science is changing every day, and it is amazing what science can tell us about ourselves in terms of current and future health.

2. *Slow down and enjoy the job.* Amazingly, when leaders recommit to what they enjoy about the job, their health improves. Superintendents need to slow down, identify priorities, and work, but not to the point of exhaustion. Your daily schedule tells a lot about your priorities. Look at your daily schedule—What items are consuming your day? What do these calendar items do to your emotional, mental, and physical health each day? No one desires to become superintendent to damage

their health. Those desires, their purpose, must be prioritized each day. Interestingly, when they are prioritized, superintendents have more time in their day, are less likely to be exhausted at the end of the day, are healthier, and have longer leadership tenures. Superintendents must work each day to make sure they are not consumed by the job—which is easy to do.

3. *Identify what you want your retirement life to look like.* If you want to have an active life during retirement, then you need to start planning now. To be clear, if you are crawling, limping, or being wheelchaired across the finish line, your retirement is not going to go the way you want it to go. Don't misconstrue what is being said. You need to give the job everything that you have, but that doesn't mean you can ruin your health and therefore what you can do after you retire. If you want to travel, then you need to make sure that you are mobile, right? Start thinking about what you want after your superintendency and make sure that your daily schedule prioritizes your health.

Voices from the Field

Preparing for Tomorrow, Today

Dr. Ruth Simpson is a sixty-five-year-old former superintendent of a suburban school district in the Northeast. As a former superintendent, Dr. Simpson completely understands what superintendents are going through. She has been retired for almost five years, but she keeps up to date on things going on in public education. When she speaks with current superintendents at conferences or with those she mentors, she is so impressed by the level of leadership that has been on display across the country to address COVID-19 over the past two years.

Over the past two years, superintendents, under new stresses and demands, have performed at levels not seen in years. She also recognizes that the pandemic has had to be emotionally, mentally, and physically draining for them and their families. Her thoughts and prayers go out to all superintendents.

The level of stress superintendents have had to endure each day and over the course of their careers is not something to overlook or take lightly. Like most superintendents, Dr. Simpson rarely focused on her health until she felt sick, her body began to ache, or she was hospitalized. Over her tenure as a superintendent, her workload landed her in the hospital for four days suffering from an irregular heartbeat and high blood pressure.

She was lucky, the physicians at the ICU told her, as she should have had a stroke by now based on her blood pressure. Her health issues and subsequent hospitalization weren't an anomaly that happened overnight. The years, months, and days before her hospitalization were physically grueling. Working eighty-plus hours a week for years made her experience health issues that could have proved deadly without some form of intervention.

Now, as Dr. Simpson approaches her fifth year of retirement, she struggles each day. Her heart continues to have irregular heartbeats from time to time, which makes her feel fatigued and have sporadic shortness of breath. She takes medication daily for her heart and high blood pressure. She finds herself having to take a lot of breaks throughout the day due to dizziness, loss of energy, and shortness of breath.

All of this restricts what she can do. She is afraid to travel too far away from her physician, and when she does, she will only take two- or three-day road trips. She has her physician on speed dial. She remains a nervous wreck those days that she travels so she prefers to stay at home—even though all she would talk about as she approached retirement was traveling abroad. Her quality of life after retirement has been diminished.

Dr. Simpson, like many superintendents, gave the job everything she had for fifteen years. She enjoyed every day, and she loved the students she was able to work with and truly had dynamic school administrators and teachers. Her only problem was that she prioritized the job and not necessarily her health. She reasoned in her head that she would focus on her health tomorrow, but she kept putting it off as something else popped up at the office.

She was too accommodating of the work schedule of day-after-day working long hours and scheduling back-to-back meetings. While she was working impossible work hours, she was neglecting her own health. Now, her health controls everything she does, from what she does each day to what she eats. Some days are better than others. Her only regret of being a superintendent is allowing the job to permanently damage her health.

If she could do it all over again, she would do so many things differently. She tells superintendents all the time not to work so hard. Like many superintendents today, Dr. Simpson was always concerned that she wasn't doing enough. Come to find out, she was working herself to physical exhaustion. Now for the rest of her life, she will be restricted in what she can do. Superintendents today have time to correct the course if they only recognize there is life after the superintendency, and if they prioritize their health and well-being today.

Key Takeaway

Superintendents have a lot of control over what happens each day in their school districts but also over their health and well-being. Many superintendents will say that the job is all-consuming, demanding so much from them emotionally, mentally, and physically. This may be true, but to have a life once a superintendent retires, they must weigh the options. They can either work themselves to an early grave or work smartly and maintain a healthy work-life balance.

No job is more important than a person's health, including a superintendent's. Superintendents must find and strike a balance between the demands of the job and their health. The superintendency requires a lot from a person, but there is some level of self-preservation that must enter the picture. No one should work to the point that they put their health in severe jeopardy. Unfortunately, the future of the superintendency will only see demands increase, but that doesn't mean that superintendents can't make fundamental shifts and prioritize their long-term health over the pressures of the job.

Conclusion

"You can't go back and change the beginning, but you can start where you are and change the ending."

—C. S. Lewis

Throughout *Prioritizing Health and Well-Being*, the message has been simple: start focusing on yourself, as superintendent, before focusing on students, teachers, and staff. Superintendents cannot effectively begin to help others with their health and well-being if their health and well-being are not taken care of. Each day, superintendents in most of the 13,000-plus school districts communicate the importance of the health and well-being to students, teachers, and staff, without ever considering their own.

Public education is witnessing an increase in superintendent burnout, exhaustion, retirement, and turnover. Due to the complexities involved with COVID-19 and cultural wars on many fronts, many equate this massive shift in the superintendency with the complexities involved with COVID-19 and the cultural wars that exist on many fronts. Maybe. But when you dive into the discussion further, superintendents are exhausted. Their social, emotional, mental, and physical health has never been worse.

Burnout and exhaustion of superintendents did not occur overnight. It has been decades in the making. If you look at many of the superintendent preparation programs, few, if any, focus on the importance of superintendent health and well-being. Likewise, few research studies exist that specifically focus on superintendent health and well-being. As the health and well-being of students and staff have hit the mainstream media and appear increasingly in research, the superintendency has been overlooked.

Superintendents have one of the most important jobs. Each superintendent is responsible for students, teachers, staff, budgets, community relations, and so many other things that consume most of their day. It is not abnormal for superintendents to work eighty-plus hours per week, Sunday through Saturday. To be clear, this workload is not sustainable for the long term. Working this hard, without any release, only leads to burnout, exhaustion, and severe health issues, as described in the "Voices from the Field" sections in each chapter.

In 2022, it is time for health and well-being to take center stage for superintendents. This is not to say that there are not superintendents already modeling the way for others when it comes to these topics, but most superintendents are not prioritizing their health and well-being. They have fallen victim to the job, which, if not moderated, will consume a person's life. Overnight, a superintendent can go from Monday through Friday, to working seven days a week. The job tends to demand everything from the superintendent, even their health and well-being.

As the beginning quote by C. S. Lewis suggests, no one can change the past, but the future can be changed. Superintendents must begin to realize that it is not only acceptable to focus on their health and well-being but also that it's a necessity of the job. Boards of education must stress to superintendents that their health and well-being must be a priority as the chief executive officer of the district. With the backing of the board of education, superintendents are more likely to accept and embrace the importance and logic of "putting their oxygen mask on first."

Superintendents, current and past, must be commended for their commitment to the job. The superintendency is often a thankless job, with most people focusing solely on something negative and little about the many positives that happen each day. As a result, stress builds up and begins to negatively impact the superintendent's health and well-being. To be effective, superintendents must be committed leaders, but there are limits to this commitment. Commitment does not mean that a superintendent's health and well-being are permanently damaged. To be clear, to be committed, a person must be healthy. To ask someone who has an unhealthy work-life balance to be committed to the job or organization is simply irresponsible and unrealistic.

Superintendents only have one mind and body. Both are irreplaceable. Once they are damaged it is extremely difficult to repair, if even possible. Instead of working like they are immortal, superintendents must recognize, before it's too late, that there are limits to what their minds and bodies can endure. Each superintendent has personalized limits. What one superintendent can take, another superintendent may not be able to. They must recognize their own limits and find ways to prioritize their health and well-being in meaningful ways.

Many will assume, mistakenly, that trimming off a couple of hours one week, or going to the gym once a week, or going on a diet will solve all their problems. Though all are moving in the right direction, health and well-being require full commitment from superintendents. They must consistently have a focus on their health and well-being, weighing the pros and cons of the job on their overall health. Maintaining a healthy work-life balance, especially as superintendents, is not easy, but it is necessary, personally and professionally.

Many superintendents will question if it is too late to focus on their health and well-being. The answer? It is never too late, though the journey back to a positive work-life balance may be more difficult for some, while less difficult for others. No matter if you are a first-year superintendent or a twenty-year veteran, if your health and well-being are not a priority each day, make them one, quickly. The sooner you recognize the importance of your health and well-being in terms of your personal and professional life, the better off you will be. Once you do, you begin to weigh the demands of the job against your health and are better equipped to find ways to reach a balance.

The best way to begin your health and well-being journey is to make it simple. Health and well-being are not complicated, but they are elusive to too many superintendents today. The best advice is to make it simple, align with your health and well-being goals and needs, and hold yourself accountable, just like you hold yourself accountable professionally. Your health and well-being are not things to take lightly, as there can be severe, and even deadly, outcomes.

If you don't know how to begin, reach out to superintendents who are modeling the way. If you don't know someone, find a physician that focuses on the health and well-being of professionals. If those two aren't options, then use the "Practical Strategies" offered in each chapter. They are good beginning points. Again, each strategy is simple and free to every superintendent who wants to begin their journey.

As you finish reading this book and you begin or resume your personal health and well-being journey, join the hundreds of superintendents on Twitter by using the hashtag #FITSupts. Changing the superintendency from one that is unhealthy for leaders to one that prioritizes health and well-being is not going to be easy. But it starts with one single person and, hopefully, that is you.

Remember, it is never too late to begin your journey; what is important is that you start. To do so, lead with understanding. Though contrary to widespread belief, it is not only acceptable but also necessary for superintendents to make their health a priority before prioritizing the health of others. No superintendent can be effective if their health and well-being are not prioritized! Though rarely discussed in research or in superintendent preparation programs, the superintendent's health and well-being are the prerequisites to becoming an effective superintendent.

Inherently Personal: A Voice from the Field

"Life is a long journey, with problems to solve, lessons to learn, but most of all, experiences to enjoy."

—Unknown

Highly effective educators become superintendents, not for the title, but for the responsibility. There is a genuine desire to serve and help others. The career of a superintendent hopefully includes many positive outcomes for students, teachers, staff, and the community. But now, in this season, when an alarming number of superintendents are leaving the profession, the goal is to help the nation's superintendents develop a healthy work-life balance.

Just like many of you who are superintendents, my well-being story is not free from setbacks, failures, and course corrections. As a former high school principal, I ended up in the emergency room due to fatigue, stress, and burnout. Working eighty-plus hours a week is not something that I am proud of or a herculean level of success that I strived to reach. Let's be honest, working this many hours a week is insane and not needed.

When I became a superintendent in 2014, the next few years, my weight ballooned up, which started creating additional issues such as chronic knee pain, regular fatigue, headaches, and, more than likely, depression, though not diagnosed. Though I was giving 100 percent to the job, I put my health on the backburner, as well as my family. Though the school district was moving forward, student achievement was improving, and operations were stabilizing, my health and well-being were rapidly declining.

Like many of you, I was raised to push through adversity and pain, but when it comes to health and well-being, this is not the best logic to adopt. I kept pushing myself in the job, working long hours, leaving work to go home to have dinner, only to leave after inhaling my food to go to school performance or athletic event. My schedule just didn't have time to squeeze in anything else that didn't pertain to the job. In my first two to three years, I was working nonstop seven days a week. I didn't have time for myself, and on the days when I somehow had free minutes or stretches of time, I still focused on the job, not my health or my daughter and wife.

I completely understand where you are and where you are heading if your health and well-being are not on your immediate radar. If you do not make the choice to focus on your health and well-being now, you will be forced at some point to focus on your health, but it may be too late. Taking the first step is always the hardest, but it is critically important. No matter if you are a novice, a veteran, approaching retirement, or an aspiring superintendent, today is the opportunity to take the first step. With that first step, you begin to build longevity not just as a superintendent but also in life.

What I have learned since prioritizing my health and well-being is that I have become a better leader, spouse, and father. At forty-one, they say my life is half over, which always makes me stop and reflect on my first forty years—what do I have to show for it? I have lived an incredibly happy, blessed, and successful life. Every day brings obstacles and setbacks, and there are some things I would change if given the opportunity. Who wouldn't? But overall, it hasn't been bad. But that does not mean the next forty is guaranteed to be just as successful if not more rewarding. As I write this, my daughter, Georgia, just turned eight years old and is in third grade. I've prioritized my health and well-being so that I am there for her and my wife, hopefully, for the next forty years.

I wrote *Prioritizing Health and Well-Being* to help superintendents discover the possibilities for their health and family by prioritizing their own health and well-being. Like with all adults, focusing on health is not the easiest journey. There are so many things to know about health and well-being, but what I have learned is *less is more*. Magazines, television, and books make health and well-being too hard and often too elusive for superintendents, or any adult for that matter. But keeping your health and well-being simple each day will not only make it possible daily but also something that can be for the long term.

Though *Prioritizing Health and Well-Being* is for all superintendents, it is a means of reflection and accountability for me. With each chapter, I offered deeply personal thoughts, a reflection of where I am with the strategy provided. I would like to tell you that I have perfected my health and well-being, but each day there are setbacks and obstacles. But there are also so many successes. I offer you an inside look at my journey to help you develop your journey to become a better superintendent by finding a positive and healthy work-life balance.

I can do this, and so can you. Our health and well-being are that important!

Afterword

Balancing professional responsibilities with our personal priorities has forever been a struggle for most every superintendent I know. While the pandemic has made it even harder for us to achieve that balance, it has also amplified the absolute need for it. And herein lies our challenge: now is the time to create that balance for ourselves. Nobody else will do it for us. Nobody else will give us the permission to prioritize health and family.

The reality is that the expectations of superintendents to be superhuman will always remain unless we change the paradigm. And the pandemic has gifted us the opportunity to do just that. *Prioritizing Health and Well-Being* reminds us that "it is mission-critical to transform the superintendency." As we reflect on what we have learned, lost, and loved during this challenging chapter in our shared history, the time is now to carve out our own healthier, more sustainable way of living and leading by focusing on six things: gratitude, persistence, endurance, grace, modeling, and perspective.

Gratitude. Actively practicing gratitude became a daily part of survival for many during the pandemic. Research is clear that practicing gratitude improves the quality of our sleep, resilience, and overall mood. Doing this has not only helped me but it has also had a very positive impact on my team. As part of our commitment to social-emotional learning, we end each of our cabinet meetings with an optimistic closure, and I often take that opportunity to share what I am grateful for and why. In times of hardship, it is easy to feel overwhelmed by the negative. Focusing on what we are grateful for pushes us, even momentarily, to stop and acknowledge all the good in our lives.

Persistence. Not perfection. Many of us in leadership arrived where we are today because of our own tendency toward perfectionism. This can be our downfall. Aspiring to perfection can prevent us from taking smart, strategic risks, and in doing so we risk never being the courageous leaders our students and communities need us to be. While we may feel tremendous pressure to be perfect, at the end of the day what people truly need and want from us is to strive to do what is right, acknowledge when we get it wrong, and persist in working to do better.

Endurance. All of us are familiar with the phrase, "This is a marathon, not a sprint," and this is certainly true in the superintendency. Our students are relying on us to remain in this work for the long haul. Giving so much of ourselves, to the point where we feel depleted or even fall ill, is not a badge of honor. COVID-19 has retaught us that staying home when we are not feeling well—physically or mentally—is necessary, which is why exercise, eating well, doing things we love with people we love is so critical. Sprinting for a couple of years in the job is not nearly as impactful as steadily making progress over seven to ten years, which is the time it takes to really achieve meaningful change in a school system.

Grace. Not guilt. The critics' voices are always the loudest and most persistent. Knowing that we will stumble at times to endure, we must fight each day to drown out those voices and find confidence in who we are and what we stand for. This means extending grace to ourselves as we do to others. It also means letting go of the guilt we often feel when we rightly choose to prioritize our own health and family. Someone once told me that guilt is a wasted emotion, so let's give ourselves guilt-free grace—especially when life is at its most challenging. Enjoy that time at your child's play, lunch with a dear friend, or time alone reading a non-education book—and do it guilt-free so that you can reap the restorative benefits of that much-needed personal time.

Modeling. One of the most powerful things we do as leaders is model. And while that modeling is most often about work ethic, professionalism, and integrity, it must also be about balance. I remember years ago worrying about anyone seeing me leave the office in my workout clothes. What would they think about my priorities? Shouldn't I be the last person pulling out of the parking lot? No! One of the best things we can do for our teams is to not simply tell them to take care of themselves but to give them permission to do so by doing it ourselves. If the superintendent can do it, so can they. The reality is that as superintendents we are always on call, so we must make time for ourselves when we can and remember that there is no cookie at the end of the day for the last person out of the parking lot.

Perspective. In the past when people asked if I love my job I would automatically and emphatically say, "Yes!" In recent years, however, I have developed a more nuanced answer. I make a distinction between the job and the work. I love my job most days but not every day. The job entails personal and professional attacks, toxicity, unrealistic expectations, and the fact that every decision we make will disappoint someone—often many someones. But the work, the work of serving children, is a gift even on the hardest of days. Keeping this perspective has been instrumental in keeping me in this work for well over a decade now. So whatever perspective helps sustain you, hold onto it tightly.

Finally, as we focus on our own individual health and well-being, let's also focus on our collective health and well-being. Never underestimate the impact that your outreach means to a fellow superintendent who is struggling or hurting. Whether you know them personally or not, send a note or email letting them know they are not alone. Reframing the superintendency in ways that allow us to remain healthy and well must also address the isolation that so many of us have felt over the years. The stronger we are, the stronger our profession will be.

Dr. Susan Enfield, superintendent
Highline Public Schools, Washington

Appendix

Below are fifteen strategies that superintendents can utilize as they begin or resume the journey to prioritize their health and well-being. They are not organized in any particular order but instead are designed to be done altogether.

1. *Put your oxygen mask on first.* Superintendents are trained to focus on everyone else first. They are trained that "leaders eat last." The thing about this is, if they are not making their own health and well-being a priority, they will not be able to help students and staff with their health and well-being. This is a time for superintendents to practice what they preach and make their health and well-being a priority.
2. *Start today.* It is never too late for superintendents to make their health and well-being a priority. Don't start tomorrow, but instead start today. Procrastination is counterproductive. Eventually, your health will make you make time, so why not make time today?
3. *Manage your calendar and schedule.* If you are not making time for yourself each day, then you negatively impact your health and well-being. Rearrange your schedule so that it allocates time for you to focus on yourself. Disconnect from technology as often as possible, whether it's email, cell phones, or social media. You will be surprised by how connected to yourself and others you will become.
4. *Don't overlook the importance of water.* You need to drink at least eight cups of water per day. It is up to you whether to drink flavored water,

just be careful about the addition of sugars and other counterproductive additives. If you can drink plain water, the better off you are, and you will notice how much better you feel.

5. *Watch your diet.* Superintendents are bad at eating on the go or whatever is available. First, schedule your lunch and try to eat at the same time each day. Everyone knows this is your protected time. Secondly, eat a healthy lunch, not fast food. Be careful of eating in cafeterias, as the food is fulfilling but loaded with calories and carbohydrates that for adults are counterproductive. Thirdly, stay away from the breakroom, vending machines, or your stash of snacks. If you must, make sure that you are purchasing healthy snacks.

6. *Walk throughout the day.* When it comes to your health, walking is transformative. Try to get your 10,000 steps each day. The best way to do so is to schedule walkthroughs in classrooms and schools. Visit classes not only to observe instruction but also to help your health. If you can schedule morning and afternoon walkthroughs do so, but if you can only do walkthroughs during a certain period, schedule right after you eat lunch. Watch how much better you feel walking each day.

7. *Get sleep.* It is extremely hard for superintendents to maintain their health and well-being with only a few hours of sleep. Sleeping at least seven hours a day is good for your immune system, weight, mental clarity, physical strength, and overall mood. If you are not sleeping enough, you are risking your health as you will see weight gains, more headaches, less energy, and so on.

8. *Exercise.* The goal is to work out at least three to four times each week. The key is to schedule your workouts, instead of squeezing in when you can. Either workout before going to work or right after work, but just do it. If you don't feel like exercising, start your exercise, and after ten minutes chances are you will continue your exercise. Exercise can be running, jogging, walking, rowing, swimming, playing a pick-up game at the YMCA, or weightlifting. The key is to move for at least forty-five minutes.

9. *Make time for yourself.* Strategically schedule at least twenty minutes each day, or multiple times throughout the day for rejuvenating. During these twenty minutes, you are reading, meditating, journaling, walking, listening to music, or just sitting in silence. No emails, no phone calls. The key is to be alone somewhere, allowing you to connect with yourself and give your mind a break.

10. *Be there for your family.* Though the pressures of the job may make you believe that you can't be there for family obligations, you can. Spending time with family is transformative for health and well-being. A superintendent cannot work twenty-four hours a day, seven days a week, and 365 days each year without a break. Attend your son's or daughter's athletic event, have dinner with your kids and wife, and spend the weekend with them. Whatever the job may demand, it can wait while you attend to your family. Get your work-life balance back into equilibrium.

11. *Hold yourself accountable.* Ideally, superintendents will have enough personal accountability to hold themselves to prioritize their health and well-being. If not, partner up with someone at the office or another superintendent for accountability. Talk, exercise together, and share with someone who can help you keep focused on your health and well-being goals.

12. *Delegate and build capacity.* Superintendents can't do everything. When they begin to believe that they have all the answers, they can be at every event, and they can be everything to everybody, that is thinking that leads to exhaustion and burnout, which is detrimental to their health and well-being. Delegate tasks to others and free up time in your schedule. As you do, you build capacity in the leaders of others while protecting your health. Superintendents are not superhuman or immortal and must begin to lead recognizing they are mortal.

13. *Don't give up.* As superintendents begin or resume their health and well-being journey, they will undoubtedly face obstacles and setbacks. The key is to jump back on the wagon and continue. Missing or skipping a workout, cheating on a diet, working long hours, or missing a family event will happen, but don't allow it to become the norm.

14. *Practice prevention, not reaction.* The more a superintendent can practice preventative care, such as eating a healthy diet, exercising, and getting enough sleep, the better off they will be when it comes to their health and well-being. Right now, too many superintendents are only addressing their health and well-being when something goes wrong. Schedule regular checkups with physicians, prioritize your schedule, and don't wait so long to seek help when there are health problems. These will help considerably.

15. *Go for long, not short yardage.* Superintendents must stop thinking about today and start looking at tomorrow and the long term when it comes to their health and well-being. If superintendents continue

working long hours, getting no sleep, eating unhealthy diets, and not taking regular breaks, their longevity as superintendents and their health and well-being will be impacted. They must put as much focus on planning for the future, in terms of their health and well-being, instead of only focusing on their health today.

Bibliography

Brunner, C. C., Grogan, M., & Bjork, L. (2002). Shifts in the discourse defining the superintendency: Historical and current foundations of the position. *The LSS Review, 1,* 22–23.

Carter, G. R., & Cunningham, W. G. (1997). *The American school superintendent: Leading in an age of pressure.* Jossey-Bass.

Glass, T., & Franceschini, L. (2007). *The state of the American school superintendency: A mid-decade study.* Rowman & Littlefield.

Kane, K. T. (2017). *Occupational stressors and job satisfaction of Pennsylvania school district superintendents* (Publication No. 10684477) [Doctoral dissertation, Widener University]. ProQuest Dissertation & Theses Global.

Kowalski, T. J. (2005). *The school superintendent: Theory, practice, and cases.* Sage.

Peterson, M. (2017). *Stress and the female superintendent: Contributing factors and stress management strategies from the voices of California female superintendents* [Doctoral dissertation, Brandman University]. https://digitalcommons.umassglobal.edu/edd_dissertations/153.

Robinson, K. & Shakeshaft, C. (2016). Superintendent stress and superintendent health: A national study. *Journal of Education and Human Development, 5*(1), 120–33. https://doi.org/10.15640/jehd.v5n1a13.

Targgart, K. T. (2017). *Stress in the superintendency* (Publication No. 10642780) [Doctoral dissertation, Ball State University]. ProQuest Dissertation & Theses Global.

Tienken, C. (Ed.). (2021). *The American superintendent: 2020 decennial study.* Rowman & Littlefield.

About the Author

Brian K. Creasman, EdD, is currently superintendent of Fleming County Schools in Kentucky. He is the 2020 Kentucky Superintendent of the Year. His Twitter account says he has the best job in Kentucky. He has served as an assistant superintendent, a high school and middle school principal and assistant principal, and an instructional technologist and classroom teacher. He is the coauthor of *The Leader Within: Understanding and Empowering Teacher Leaders*; *Growing Leaders Within: A Process toward Teacher Leadership*; *Can Every School Succeed? Bending Constructs to Transform an American Icon*; *ConnectED Leaders: Network and Amplify your Superintendency*; and *Maximum Impact: Boards of Education and Superintendents Communicating as a Team*. Brian can be reached at briankcreasman@gmail.com. He can also be found on Twitter at @FCSSuper. He is the founder of #FITSupts and is co-moderator of #bendingED, the national and international school transformation chat on Twitter.

www.ingramcontent.com/pod-product-compliance
Lightning Source LLC
Chambersburg PA
CBHW022318280326
41932CB00010B/1145